The Practical Guide to Toilet Training Your Child with Low Muscle Tone

Sensory-Motor Secrets for Success

Cathy Collyer, OTR, LMT

Cathy Collyer, OTR, LMT

Also by the Author

The JointSmart Child: Living and Thriving with Hypermobility Volume One: The Early Years

The JointSmart Child: Living and Thriving with Hypermobility Volume Two: The School Years

The Practical Guide to Toilet Training the Autistic Child: Sensory-Motor Secrets for Success

The Practical Guide to Toilet Training Your Child with Low Muscle Tone, second edition

August 1, 2023
Written and published by CathyAnn Collyer, OTR, LMT

tranquilbabies.com

Version 2.0 © 2023 CathyAnn Collyer
All rights reserved

Disclaimer:

The information contained in this book is based on the author's experience, knowledge, and opinions. It is not a replacement for clinical evaluation and treatment. The author and publisher will not be held liable for the use or misuse of the information in this book.

Special thanks to Laurie Dubner and Vivian Kahn Adler, who have been amazing team members in my clinical work with children with low muscle tone. Thanks as well to Edward Matte, whose technical assistance has been invaluable. Most importantly, warmest regards and grateful thanks to all the families of children with low muscle tone who have welcomed my support as they go on their potty training journey; you have taught me more than I have taught you!

Cathy Collyer, OTR, LMT

The Practical Guide to Toilet Training Your Child with Low Muscle Tone

Section I   The Basics

Section II   The Magic of Targeted Pre-Training

Section III   Time to Train: The Rubber Meets the Road

The Practical Guide to Toilet Training Your Child with Low Muscle Tone

- *Are you wondering if a child is ready for toilet training?*
- *Has their developmental pediatrician suggested that it is time to start training?*
- *Are you hoping that school will do the majority of their training?*
- *Have you repeatedly run into problems during potty training?*
- *Do you wonder what the right potty seat or clothes are?*
- *Are speech or sensory delays issues?*
- *Are you a teacher or therapist, responsible for toilet training at school?*
- *Do you need strategies to improve safety and coordination?*

This book is for parents who want to help children with low tone learn to use the toilet, but don't understand why it is so challenging, or what to do differently.
This book is also for the therapists and teachers who want to do toilet training at school or in a clinic and wish to support the families of the children in their care.

This is a practical guide that prepares children for success.

I have been a pediatric occupational therapist for over 25 years. Helping children with low muscle tone achieve skills that seemed out of reach, and seeing them grow and thrive, has been amazing. Some families have asked me for direct instruction in toilet training strategies and for advice on adaptive equipment.

Many others have not.

They incorrectly assumed that my professional skill set was limited to addressing sensory processing or improving handwriting. It is not always clear to families or other professionals that experienced occupational therapists have the wide breadth and depth of knowledge that can help their child achieve toileting independence. As an occupational therapist, I am the member of the therapy team that pulls together my understanding of neuroscience, psychology, physiology, and task analysis to help children learn independent living skills. As a home-care therapist for Early Intervention programs, and as a therapist in private practice, I have spent many years working directly with families in their homes. They and their children have taught me more than I have taught them. Their wisdom and insights are in every page of this book. If a parent feels that they are alone on this journey, they should know that there are many parents just like them, trying their best every day and looking for answers. Some of the answers they seek are right here, in this book.

If a teacher or therapist feels that they are struggling to understand why families aren't as responsive to strategies or eager to buy and use adaptive equipment, this book offers them some insight and additional techniques to work with a family's concerns and motivations to get great results. Self-care skills such as toileting might appear less important to a hypotonic child's development than speech or mobility skills. This is understandable; there is a strong hope that things as simple as getting dressed and using the toilet will naturally emerge when a child is walking and talking.

This is short-sighted. Self-care skills do more than create independence in activities of daily living (ADLs). I believe that the acquisition of essential independent living skills such as toileting are pivotal to developing a child's self-esteem and their sense of agency in their world. Taking care of everyday personal needs allows a child to separate their actions and identity from those of their caregivers. This occurs without a child being able to define self-esteem. We see the change almost immediately after they say, "I did it!" Feeling more empowered and confident is visible in the new ways they move through their world. Performing self-feeding, dressing, and toileting all require the use of focused attention, sensory processing, communication, and social skills. These abilities are applied for a practical purpose, with a visible end point in mind. Children develop the ability to think logically and flexibly in the moment when they perform self-care skills. They see the tangible (and measurable!) results of their physical effort.

Learning to use the toilet independently has meaning, it has memory, and it changes a child's life.

After reviewing books on toileting, I realized that most chapters on toilet training children with low tone rarely provided detailed answers and full explanations. The authors that provided great training strategies did not always explain why these worked or told parents what to do if their methods failed. Children with low muscle tone don't face the same issues as other children with different developmental challenges, and they are rarely the focus of chapters on "special needs" toilet training. They don't have the same issues with attention and interpersonal skills that kids on the autistic spectrum face, nor do they have a need for specialized equipment like many children with cerebral palsy. Children with low tone aren't necessarily defiant, or always sensory-sensitive. Over time, it became clear to me that no one was giving parents of young children with low muscle tone the comprehensive support for toilet training they needed to be successful.

I believe the primary issue many adults and almost all children encounter in potty training is that neither party has adequate preparation to begin training. Things get started, and inevitably, problems ensue. They do not know why things have gone off the rails or how to get training back on track. This book assists parents and professionals in determining if they and the child are ready for training. If a child is not yet 18 months-old, or if they have major developmental delays... their family and caregivers need this book even more than the child who is fully ready to train, because I teach them to pre-train! In my experience, the parents and caregivers of children who consistently use pre-training strategies before they start formal training see faster toilet training progress. They have fewer surprises, and there is less guesswork, pausing of training, and frustration on everyone's part. Training, and life, gets easier for everyone.

Why is toilet training so important?

One way to stay focused and positive on this journey is to remember why children need to be toilet trained. All children need to learn to use the toilet, unless their cognitive or medical issues make it impossible. It is the easiest, quickest, and cleanest way to deal with urination and bowel movements. But there are other practical reasons. Independent elimination into a toilet allows children to engage in academic and social activities that would otherwise not be available to them. Most integrated classrooms and integrated sports or music activities must make significant accommodations for an incontinent child. At the minimum they may require an outside adult to be available for diaper changes.

There are medical reasons that kids with low muscle tone need to learn to use the toilet instead of diapers. Children who wear diapers are at risk for chronic diaper rash. This is more than inconvenient or unsightly. Once the skin of the buttocks and genital area has been irritated, it is susceptible to recurrent irritation or infection. The use of prolonged courses of prescription cortisone cream thins and weakens the skin, making it even more fragile and vulnerable. Seeing a child in pain and seeing their red, raised skin is very difficult for most adults. It turns an otherwise healthy child into a child that is seen as medically fragile. Their refusal to remain seated isn't always connected to their diaper rash, because the providers interacting with children are not necessarily aware of the problem. These kids are seen as being oppositional or even hyperactive. They are nothing of the kind; their bottom is too sore to sit on! Eliminating the risk of chronic diaper rash is a terrific reason to work toward toileting independence.

Another important consideration is the decreased risk of sexual abuse. Sadly, abuse happens more often in the same locations and by the same people that abuse neurotypical children. Kids with special needs are abused by people they know well. It happens in their home, or in the homes of their relatives and close family friends. Occasionally it occurs in a day program. A child that can use the bathroom independently is far less vulnerable to sexual abuse than a child that needs an adult to touch their genitals for care that occurs in a private location.

How is this book different from the dozens of "special needs toileting" books on the market?

That is simple: it is in the title. This is a <u>practical</u> guide to toilet training. It isn't a book that is theory-heavy and light on useful ideas. There are a wide variety of skills taught during potty training. These skills include everything an adult does from the moment they know they need to use the toilet. Taken together, they demonstrate a very simple fact about toilet training:

Using the toilet isn't primarily a behavioral skill. It is a sensory-motor self-care skill that has behavioral components.

This book focuses on the unique needs of kids with low muscle tone, also known as hypotonia. These terms will be interchangeable throughout every chapter. Many different medical diagnoses include hypotonia, because it is a symptom, not a disorder. It used to be that kids would be labeled as having "idiopathic hypotonia", which is loosely translated as "We don't know why this is happening, but it is." With the onset of whole genome testing, many of the children that would be placed in the category of "idiopathic hypotonia" are now being identified as having genetic disorders. While parents often experience acute shock when told that their child has a genetic disorder, almost every family finds that getting an answer, and connecting with other parents of similarly diagnosed kids, makes their lives easier. I encourage families to join support groups and pursue skilled therapies that can make a difference for their child.

Children with low tone don't face the same blend of toilet training issues as children with other developmental challenges. They and their families <u>deserve</u> their own manual. It is common for an autistic child to have low muscle tone and to have limited hand coordination. It is common to see kids with ADHD to have sensory processing issues. Hypotonia is rarely the primary challenge for autistic kids or hyperactive kids. Their most common reasons for delayed toileting independence are different. Not always more intense, but different. Kids with low muscle tone have specific social and emotional challenges that stem from their challenges in development. Their sensory processing problems can be more complex than those of other special needs kids. This is true both for the intensity of their sensory struggles and the many types of sensory processing they find difficult to perform. A child that both seeks and avoids sensory experiences, while being insensitive to other sensations will require a different approach than a child who only displays sensory sensitivity. Hypotonic children may need adaptive equipment to be successful in toileting. They will not need the same equipment or use equipment in the same manner as a child with cerebral palsy.

There are other differences between this book and many books on toilet training the special needs child. There are no record-keeping charts in this book. Why? Because parents do not use them for very long, and they often need a behaviorist to help them translate the chart into meaningful information. Very few parents and teachers have the time and energy for this. They are scrambling just to get through the day! Asking busy parents to start a project that will ultimately frustrate them or fill them with guilt and discouragement, that they abandon shortly after starting it, is not helpful. They can learn a great deal through other observational methods; methods that don't tax them in the same way. This book covers ALL the skills involved in using the toilet. Peeing and pooping into the toilet isn't the end of training. Clothing management, flushing, and washing and drying hands are all necessary to get the job completely done.

The Adults Doing the Training Need Support Too!

A review of books on special needs toilet training indicated that no one was giving the parents, caregivers, and teachers of autistic children enough information and emotional support through the toilet training process to ensure success. There is more to this book than teaching the steps of toilet training. Anyone raising, teaching, or treating autistic children knows that this is demanding work. Even when it is done with love, it is still a lot of mental and physical work. There are new problems and new complications coming at parents and professionals every day. All day. Every day. This book is specifically designed to offer support to the adults raising and working with hypotonic children. It focuses on practical ideas that make a visible difference. This inspires them to keep going. Parents and professionals can go to an IEP meeting armed with information they can use to develop a better plan and help write next year's goals. That is empowerment.

Using the toilet is an essential life skill, and it is a life skill that has historically been linked with feelings of shame around elimination. That makes everyone's feelings about potty training tricky to unpack. Most kids have far less shame about elimination than the adults that are helping them. Because toilet training involves touching and viewing genitals, many adults are uncomfortable answering the questions children raise or using the anatomical words for body parts. There can be a lot of shame around parenting a child who engages in smearing behaviors, who has elimination accidents in public, or who smells bad because they refuse to allow diaper changes or don't wipe their body well after toileting. Caregivers may think that it is their job to prevent all accidents, when in fact, accidents are important learning opportunities for the child and their team.

This book doesn't ignore or minimize any of this complexity. It tackles it head-on. All this effort and emotion can shrink an adult's mental bandwidth. It makes them prone to getting discouraged, worried, and frustrated. Adults doing toilet training with kids low muscle tone need emotional support and simple explanations of useful strategies.

Potty Stories

This book has a unique writing style; it combines practical explanations of pre-training and formal toilet training with narrative accounts of three fictional families working on toilet training their child. These are completely fictional accounts, drawn from decades of experience with children, families, and teachers. Illustrating what it looks, sounds, and feels like to toilet train children by telling a story is helpful for readers with non-linear learning styles. It is also helpful for readers whose big emotions play a large part of the struggles they have during potty training. Painting a picture can be more

11

powerful than making a to-do list. Narratives combined with facts simply help the brain learn quickly and easily. Recognizing the emotional and social issues surrounding potty training is important for everyone, and narratives express feelings in a way that behavioral plans do not. Adults with lots of frustration, fear, or anxiety around toilet training will find that they resonate with character's struggles more than with a list of strategies or suggestions. Solutions and strategies become easier to appreciate when the emotions around toilet training are embraced, not hidden.

Let's meet our families:

Family One:

Tiffany and Corey have two children. Olivia is their youngest. She is 18 months old, with a fiercely independent streak and lots of language. She loves her puppy and cuddling in bed with her parents. James is 3 and was diagnosed with HADDS shortly before his second birthday. James is non-verbal but can use a few signs. He has many issues with sensory processing that make going to his self-contained class more challenging. He resists being held and helped with meals and bathing.

Jacqueline, Tiffany's mom, watches Olivia during the day and James after he comes home from school. Tiffany describes her mom's approach to childcare as "old school". Jacqueline understands that spanking isn't OK, but she can be harsh when her grandchildren don't listen to her. She thinks that her daughter and son-in-law should have already been potty training both kids, as she got all three of her children "day-trained" by 2. James's primary teacher is Zulema. She is enthusiastic about doing toilet training at school. She is a fairly new teacher, and she has two great teacher aides in her classroom.

Family Two:

Sean and Luke are married and have one daughter, Bella. She was conceived using a surrogate and Sean's sperm. Bella is 8; she has never developed any verbal skills. Her mild epilepsy is well-controlled by medication now. Whole genome testing identified alterations in DNA but no definitive diagnosis. Bella needs help for all of her personal care. While she has no verbal language, and she will self-injure at times when she is very upset, she has recently learned a few signs. She is generally floppy. Walking took her until she was 3, and she still isn't running or climbing stairs by alternating her feet. Bella is showing her dads that she wants her diaper changed soon after she soils it. A wet diaper doesn't seem to bother her. She rarely indicates that she needs anything other than one of her dad's phones or iPads.

Padriac and Maggie are Luke's parents. They live locally, and care for Bella after school at their house. Padriac and Maggie are originally from Ireland. They raised Luke and his sisters in America. Maggie remembers training Luke as a toddler after using only cloth diapers. She is against the idea of using what she calls "plastic" diapers and training pants. Sima is Bella's occupational therapist at the outpatient clinic she attends 3x/week. Sima has considerable experience with toilet training. She is an Israeli immigrant. Maggie often has a very difficult time understanding Sima's English when they discuss Bella's progress, but she is embarrassed to mention this to anyone but her husband.

Family Three:
Jordan and Lewis divorced shortly after Henry's birth. Jordan already had a child, Simone, from her first marriage. They have two kids together: Angela and Henry. Angela is a gifted 10-year old with a passion for soccer. Henry is 4 and has a diagnosis of idiopathic hypotonia. Jordan and Lewis knew that his development was slow, but their pediatrician kept assuring them that he would catch up. That has not happened, and now Henry is in an integrated preschool program in their school district. Simone's ADHD has taken a back seat to Henry's needs. Jordan's guilt keeps her up at night far too often, but she feels pulled in about 100 directions. Jordan has a live-out nanny, Danielle. Danielle raised 6 kids of her own as a single mother. Without Danielle, Jordan is certain she would be on psychiatric meds or drink more wine than she already does! She knows that Danielle has her own ideas about potty training, and she is worried that they will conflict with hers or her therapy team's ideas.

Lewis has the two youngest kids at his apartment on alternate weekends and school holidays. His mom, Sharon, is in town for the summer, but lives in Florida the rest of the year. Sharon is a retired special education teacher. Jordan thinks her ex mother-in-law tries to present herself as the ultimate authority on <u>anything</u>

to do with special needs education. Lewis doesn't like conflict with anyone, so he rarely contradicts his mother when she decides to "educate" everyone. Sharon thinks she could potty train Henry in a week if they would only let her.

What's Inside?

Section I: The Basics

These chapters describe why toilet training hypotonic children can be different from standard toilet training, how to spot readiness in these kids, and how digestive difficulties can derail the best potty training strategies. Some of the differences in training are obvious to everyone, and some are a surprise to even experienced parents and professionals. Without knowing this territory in detail, it is harder to be prepared. Many adults are unsure about what the signs of readiness really are when a child has low tone and significant functional delays. The goalposts might seem to change with the day if readiness signs aren't clear to everyone. It is worth mentioning that only some of the readiness signs are *child* readiness. The home or school needs to be ready with equipment, finances, and more. The adults involved need to be ready and informed about the territory ahead.

Section II: The Magic of Targeted Pre-Training

The magic of pre-training is explained in detail. Targeted pre-training builds skills and confidence in both the child being trained *and* the adults teaching and supervising. Much of the pre-training happens while the child is still wearing diapers all day. Transitioning from being passively diapered to being part of the experience of elimination into a toilet or potty seat is a process. Pre-training is essential for hypotonic children of all ages and at all levels of ability. It is magic. Really.

Section III: Time to Train: The Rubber Meets the Road

Formal training requires a good plan and the ability to flex and pivot. Whether using the gradual approach or the "potty intensive", knowing what makes formal training successful is important. Being fully trained means a child can independently use *any* toilet in *any* location. This isn't always easy for hypotonic kids. Their delays in movement, communication, and sensory processing issues alone can be more than enough to make using the public toilet harder, scarier, and less desirable. We see defiance, withholding, true fear responses, and more. Knowing how to navigate through all of these is just as important as doing a good job of pre-training. Getting all the way to this final point in the journey requires creativity, confidence, and conviction. These chapters help families, caregivers, teachers, and therapists craft a plan and adjust it along the way.

How to Use This Book

As a practical guide this book can be used in many ways:

1. *To prepare families and caregivers for potty training at every stage, all the way to full independence.*
2. *To teach great toilet training strategies to new teachers or therapists, or to teach seasoned professionals who are new to working with hypotonic kids.*
3. *To support a family member or babysitter who is training a child and needs more support and information.*
4. *To restart toilet training after a pause or a failure, armed with greater comprehension and a new perspective on potty training.*

Using WOOP to create Independent Toileting

There are many psychological and behavioral strategies that could be helpful when potty training a child. Potty training is a complex skill for both adults and children alike. The adults involved may never have trained a child. Ever. While this book focuses on helping adults teach children how to use the toilet, they may need help to create a laser focus and sustain their motivation. One of the most researched but simplest approaches to grappling with challenging goals is called **WOOP**.

Cathy Collyer, OTR, LMT

Gabriele Oettingen PhD has created an amazing process to meet the challenges in life with a scientific strategy that supercharges motivation and action. Her WOOP method uses something called mental contrasting. Our grandmothers would call it "being realistic", but it is much more than simply accepting the challenges in life. Dr. Oettingen uses *mental contrasting* to help people more clearly see what is holding them back, and then get them to focus on taking action to address these issues. She has spent decades proving, with repeated scientific studies, that visualizing both the obstacles that could appear as well as specific goals create meaningful subconscious patterns that make it <u>easier</u> to succeed, not harder.

I encourage anyone that is curious about WOOP to read Dr. Oettingen's book, and download her free WOOP app.

My message to every family or professional that is thinking of toilet training a child who has low muscle tone, regardless of the child's age or their level of challenge, is this:

Be well prepared, be consistent, expect to need to practice in order to make progress,
and stay positive.

You can do it!

Chapter 1

How Low Muscle Tone Creates Toilet Training Challenge

What aspects of toilet training are universal?

A child with low muscle tone is more like typically developing children than most people around them think. A history of struggles to achieve developmental milestones will, at times, make it harder for everyone to recognize a child's strengths. This can happen as easily in teachers and therapists as it can in immediate family. That is a shame; making progress in toilet training requires optimizing strengths as well as managing needs.

Using the toilet is a new and complex skill for every child. Careful adult observation, sufficient exposure to targeted practice, effective rewards, and moving independence from the home into the community are required for every child to be successfully toilet trained. The parents of kids with low muscle tone have a lot in common with their relatives and friends who are training their typically developing children. Other families get frustrated and discouraged too. They wonder if they chose the wrong time to try, or if they don't have what it takes. They celebrate successes and dream about what full independence would look like.

Toileting independence has the same larger meaning for every child: it is another step away from infancy, toward independence, and a move toward more personal freedom. Neither the child or the parents may be aware of it at the time, but independent toileting changes both how a child experiences life, and how the adults around them see their roles in relationship to the child. Parents and caretakers aren't just losing the time, mess, and expense of diapers; they have yielded control over a major physical process to the child. The potty-trained child is now in charge of their body in a powerful new way. Some parents and caregivers admit that they feel a bit wistful for the personal satisfaction of performing personal care. They liked how it felt to be needed in such an important practical way. A child's emerging independence makes them wonder what their new role will look like. This is rarely said out loud, but it should be. It is an understandable feeling that should be addressed to prevent a child from questioning their pride in the hard-won accomplishment of using the toilet alone.

Some adults recognize that getting things done around the house (or school) with a child who has just learned to use the toilet is more work than a quick diaper change. Paying attention to a toileting schedule, reminding them to use the bathroom, and supervising those early attempts at wiping and flushing take more time than diapering. I have met plenty of parents that were hoping that if they waited long enough, they could go through a weekend "potty intensive"; their child would emerge completely independent. This *does* happen. It is rare, unfortunately, because so many kids and parents must overcome the effects of years of inattention and weak skills before they do formal training. More often than not, families that waited too long to train are battling rigid habits and a child who no longer responds easily to praise and rewards.

Why potty training might be easier than expected

Even though few kids can describe the *future* benefits of using the toilet independently, they might be able to see some of the benefits to them in the moment. It is worth a parent or caregiver telling them about some of the advantages. And repeating them occasionally, when a good opportunity arises. Getting a positive reaction from a child isn't required for beneficial effects. Anyone who has raised teenagers knows that rejection of information does not mean that the information didn't sink in.

What are the advantages for a hypotonic child of being fully toilet trained?

Building self-care skill independence removes the stress of having to communicate needs to an adult and wait to receive help. If a child can satisfy their needs independently, there is no waiting, no confusion about what type and level of assistance is desired, and no frustration when the adult's actions aren't done well or in the ways that the child expects. Using the toilet rather than a diaper means no unwanted physical contact, and no remaining wet or soiled. Most typically developing children develop a dislike of having their diaper changed well before they learn to use the toilet independently. Toilet training is their opportunity to be rid of being moved, wiped, and moved around again on another person's schedule. By the age of 2, most children can be actively engaged in play for 20 minutes or more at a time. They don't want their play interrupted by another person. When they are toilet trained, they can time bathroom visits to keep playing or interrupt play at a better time. They can choose the bathroom they like best. It might be the one closest to their bedroom, or the small one with the lights that dim, or the one with the most comfortable potty insert. Or the quietest one.

When thinking about why a child is resistant to diaper changing, it is important for any caregiver to make the effort to empathize. This reduces caregiver frustration and increases the use of adaptive strategies that increase the child's participation. Any adult that has been hospitalized and needed to obtain assistance to use a bedpan or to walk to the toilet can relate to the desire to be free of needing assistance and having to follow someone else's schedule for using the bathroom. Many children find that being alone in the bathroom considerably decreases their stress around potty use. Being able to use the toilet alone places the pace and location of touch, sound, and movement in the hands of the child. Hypotonic kids often require physical assistance more frequently throughout their day, and this goes on for a longer time than typically developing kids. Privacy is an underappreciated experience. As above, any adult that has been hospitalized can tell you how relieved they are to get home and have more privacy in the bathroom. Hypotonic kids may have such limited opportunities for privacy that they often need to be shown what it feels like and hear why this is something adults find so desirable.

What aspects of hypotonia impact toilet training?

Hypotonia will almost always create challenges during toilet training. Many parents and professionals are surprised to learn that the degree of low tone may not correlate with the degree of difficulty experienced when learning to use the toilet. This is because the specific environment, the skills of a child's caregiver or therapist, and a child's age while training all impact their progress. A child's treatment team may have already identified some of the challenges ahead. They may not have shared this information widely enough. Adding to the complications, not all providers are experienced in toilet training. They also may not consider their practice sphere to extend into self-care skills. Parents and teachers that have not had consistent or extended contact with a child's therapists should ask for their direct support in developing the toilet training plan. This could save time, money, and more than a few tears! Low muscle tone is not a diagnosis; it is a symptom. Some children have been diagnosed around the time of birth with a condition in which low muscle tone is one of the diagnostic criteria. For example, all children with Down or Prader-Willi syndromes are hypotonic at birth. Many doctors will use the term "idiopathic" when they are not able to identify the cause of hypotonia in a child. This doesn't mean that a later diagnosis is not possible. With other kids, low tone is only identified as the child struggles to walk, talk, or reach other physical milestones. Some hypotonic children have minimal-to-moderate delays in their motor development. They demonstrate otherwise typical progression of cognitive, language and social skills. Others will have global delays, and work very hard to master every skill.

The hypotonic child's potential challenges can be divided into three categories: physical, sensory processing, and social/emotional issues:

Physical challenges

Children with low muscle tone either have some difficulty controlling their movements or they show more rapid fatigue than other children. Often both. A child who is not walking is not ready for formal toilet training. They will not be able to crawl fast enough to the toilet or potty seat to be consistently successful. The most common issues encountered in toilet training the hypotonic child are limited physical stability, reduced abdominal strength, and easily predictable comfortable bowel movements.

Limited Stability

Controlled stable and safe movements while sitting and standing are essential for independently using the bathroom. Elimination (the purely physical acts of peeing and pooping) requires a child to sit comfortably to relax and release those muscles controlling elimination. A child who learns to urinate in standing requires even more physical stability, more awareness of their body position, and more ability to control body movements to aim their urine stream. Managing clothing while standing, then wiping and flushing the toilet, also requires good balance while being able to look down and around the room. Without a stable sitting or standing posture, it is very difficult to feel safe and calm, and a child who is anxious can't pay sufficient attention to managing clothing, wiping, or flushing. The child must be able to relax the external sphincter muscles to release. This issue alone can result in the refusal to sit on the toilet, or a preference to eliminate into a diaper instead.

Low muscle tone limits a child's postural stability against gravity. These children often stand and sit with less control and less ability to shift their balance smoothly. Sequencing movements and performing more than one action at a time can be very difficult for the hypotonic child. Some hypotonic children will lean against any available surface or lean on one arm, leaving only one hand available for use. This isn't functional; one-handed dressing strategies are just about impossible for most children who otherwise have the use of both hands. When elimination urgency is sensed, actions need to be rapid and correctly sequenced to avoid accidents. Inefficient movements created by instability use excessive energy and time. This contributes to rapid fatigue, sometimes shocking both the caregiver and the child. A child could get to the bathroom and get on the toilet, only to practically fall of it after sitting for 5 minutes! One of the most valuable benefits of occupational therapy can be identifying all of the adaptations that rapidly increase endurance without waiting for an exercise program to build muscle strength.

To have effective vestibular processing for good balance, a typical child moves their head out of a vertical, midline orientation with sufficient frequency, intensity and within the full range available every day. This develops best when a child can move against gravity, as in sitting, standing, walking, and running. Many hypotonic kids developed these skills slowly. Some do not have them when they are otherwise ready for toilet training. Without the ability to play with balance, a child is at a disadvantage. What does "playing with balance" look like? A baby that rolls across the room to get her rattle. An older infant that bear-crawls (hands on the floor, behind up in the air) and flips over, laughing hysterically. A toddler that stands up and spins around until she falls on the floor giggling. A preschooler that walks along the curb in a heel-to-toe pattern, just because it is fun to try not to fall off the edge. Children with hypotonia may have tried to copy their siblings and peers in these ways, but often not frequently enough, with graded control, and not in time for potty training. Many become happier sitting or lying down. Gravity isn't challenging them as much. They learn to create play schemas that entertain without having to work so hard. A child that prefers to sit throughout the day is less likely to have refined balance when they get up to go to the bathroom in a hurry.

Henry had always been a floppy baby, and at 3 he was now a floppy preschooler. His dad wished he could take Henry to the park and play catch, but since Henry rarely caught a ball of any size, that wasn't going to happen. They started giving him prune juice mixed with apple juice to regulate his bowel movements in infancy. The fits he would throw when constipated meant that both Jordan and Lewis kept a 6-month supply of both juices in their homes. They felt they might never be without the "magic juice" that kept Henry regular. They worried about what would happen when/if it stopped working, or he decided that he wouldn't drink it any longer.

Chronic constipation and diarrhea are more than uncomfortable for children.

Painfully passing feces or having uncontrolled bowel movements creates fear. Chapter 3 goes into detail about the ways in which diet, digestion, and medications can either solve or contribute to problems with potty training. *Constipation* and diarrhea have many causes, and not every child with low muscle tone gets constipated or has chronic constipation. The primary contributors to constipation for children with low muscle tone are dietary issues and low abdominal muscle tone combined with low activity levels. Low muscle tone is seen in the muscles of the core and the mouth and throat. The smooth muscles that line the intestines and can be hypotonic as well.

Children can have difficulty chewing, swallowing, or coordinating the suck-swallow-breathe synchrony right from birth. This synchrony is the largely unconscious pattern we all use to toggle between eating or drinking and breathing. It is an essential skill. Without it, children can struggle with chewing, swallowing, restricting their diet, and breathing food into their lungs. Poorly chewed food, frequent choking, and actively avoiding challenging food textures that contain fiber are frequent contributors to chronic constipation and diarrhea. This can create a preference for a low-fiber diet that often contributes to constipation. A preference for foods like bananas and vegetable purees over whole foods are two examples. Difficulties with swallowing or excessive drooling can make it harder for children to stay well hydrated. Without adequate hydration, urinary infections are more common, skin is more fragile, and bowel movements become slower and harder. All of these are common in hypotonic kids, and these issues directly impact toilet training.

We also see issues with anxiety and endurance when a child's breathing is restricted in any way. This is usually related to the effort needed to use secondary breathing muscles and the effects of shallow respiration on the autonomic nervous system. This subtle stressor may only be noticed by a skilled therapist or a very observant caregiver. Our current healthcare system and our educational system has increased attention on emotional regulation but often overlooks the contribution of physical issues to a child's mental state. This is true even in a child with a clear diagnosis of hypotonia. Not treating all every cause of a child's distress leaves them more vulnerable to the inherent challenge of learning this new skill.

Smoothly Controlled Elimination

Elimination is supported by two physical events. The first is the contraction of smooth muscles in the intestines or bladder, along with the resting pressure of the abdominal muscles against these structures. This isn't done consciously. Low muscle tone and muscle weakness diminishes both. The gastro-colic reflex is present from birth; it is an internal reflex that contributes to regular bowel movements. As food enters the stomach, the stretching of the stomach wall and the entrance of food into the small intestine stimulates contraction of the small and large intestines. Muscular contraction eventually moves food in the direction of the colon for elimination. Any conditions that limit smooth muscle contraction will therefore affect intestinal motility. Low muscle tone is one of those conditions.

The second event is the creation of intra-abdominal pressure from active "bearing down" during elimination. Reduced abdominal muscle strength and low tone at rest limits the amount of stimulation the intestines and bladder receive from the abdominal wall. Low muscle tone creates a situation where children frequently have lower overall levels of activity compared with their peers. They are more likely sitting or even lying down for longer periods of the day than other kids at every age. When children are moving around, they sustain high levels of activity for shorter periods. All of this reduces the amount of active muscle contraction against the intestines throughout the day. Weaker muscles have less power to help with elimination when nature calls.

The act of intentionally increasing pressure within the abdominal cavity to assist with evacuating the colon is called the Valsalva maneuver. To use the Valsalva maneuver, a child must be able to sit on the toilet slightly forward, with knees a bit higher than hips, and contract the abdominal muscles. This is usually paired with exhaling. Children with very low tone and limited core strength find that achieving adequate postural stability <u>while</u> achieving enough intra-abdominal pressure to use the Valsalva maneuver can be difficult.

Sensory processing challenges

Children without the ability to sense the need to use the toilet and take effective physical actions will not be completely independent. Their caregivers will use scheduled eating/drinking and bathroom use to reduce bathroom accidents, but humans aren't machines. These kids will have many accidents over the course of a week. Physical skills matter as much as sensory processing. Sensing the need to eliminate but being unable to get to the toilet, manipulate clothing efficiently, sit or stand safely, and wipe/wash following elimination will prevent a child from being able to use the toilet independently.

Using the toilet, therefore, is a sensory-motor skill.

The idea that behavioral strategies build sensory and motor skills misleads families and professionals.

The importance of sensory processing on toilet training is rarely addressed in most books on special needs toilet training. It is assumed that this system is functioning effectively in the background. The assumption is that a child learns the meaning of the sensations they have, and makes the correct responses at the right time, in enough time to prevent an accident.

If a child has low muscle tone, they experience a degree of sensory processing challenge due to the interplay of tone, movement, and sensory feedback loops. Low muscle tone **always** affects a child's sensory processing to some degree. This is because hypotonia will decrease the amount and speed of information sent to the brain and create some degree of delayed response.

Cathy Collyer, OTR, LMT

Not every hypotonic child has severe enough sensory processing issues that they impact toilet training. Sensory processing problems of all types can be overcome with more experience, better training, targeted compensation, and the right equipment.

Sensory registration

When muscles contract, completely unseen events happen. Sensors within the muscles, in the surrounding fascia, in ligaments and tendons, and sensors within the joint itself register changes in length, amplitude and of force, speed and direction of movements. These sensors send this information to the brain for interpretation and possibly for action. This is proprioception and kinesthesia. The result may be movement, additional muscle activation, or quiet monitoring. Stronger contraction=more sensors activated= more signal to the brain for processing. Low muscle tone reduces the number of muscle and fascial fibers activated at rest, ready to respond for activity, and slightly slows the speed at which initial contractions occur. Fewer sensors firing and slower firing of previously inactive receptors reduce information volume and to the brain.

The ability to sense internal state and changes in state is referred to as interoception.
Managing changes in body temperature, monitoring the need for oxygen, and controlling heart rate are not under conscious control. Our autonomic nervous system manages these functions. Sensing and then responding to hunger, thirst, and elimination urgency are under our conscious control. This control is dependent on sufficient and speedy sensory feedback and correct interpretation of this information. For continence, proprioception melds with interoception as kids feel the downward pressure of a full bladder or a full rectum. The external sphincters for both the bladder and the rectum are muscles that children can learn to control during toilet training. These are what they use to "hold it" until they get to the potty. If the smooth muscles of the bladder or the skeletal muscles of the abdominal wall don't send correct information to be interpreted, then it is much harder for a child to be continent.

Children with poor interoceptive and proprioceptive awareness frequently deny that they need to use the toilet and they could refuse to try if their trainers don't understand this issue. The puddle under their chair or their mad dash to the bathroom suggests that these kids weren't lying; they really didn't get the sensory messages clearly and promptly.

Good vestibular processing while sitting and standing are very, very important for using the toilet safely. A child needs to sit comfortably to sufficiently relax and allow elimination to occur. A boy who urinates in standing requires even more stability, positional awareness, and carefully controlled movements to aim his urine stream into the toilet or urinal. Managing clothing while standing, then wiping and flushing, are some other complex toileting skills that require good balance while looking down and looking around. To develop the level of effective vestibular processing needed for good balance, a child must move their head out of a vertical, midline orientation with sufficient frequency, intensity and within the full range available every day. Over time, balance is effortless and carefully graded. Slight changes in position don't provoke large reactions.

What does that look like? A baby that rolls across the room to get her rattle. An infant that bear-crawls (hands on the floor, behind up in the air) and flips over into their caregiver's arms. A toddler that stands up and spins around until she falls on the floor giggling. A preschooler walking along the curb in a heel-to-toe pattern because it is fun for them to try to stay along the edge. Children with low tone have done some or most of these things, but often not frequently enough and not at the same stage as their same-age peers. Issues with posture and balance that contribute to delayed walking can also delay toileting readiness.

Kids with low muscle tone may have sensory processing issues other than limited registration. These further complicate learning complex functional skills like toilet training. Skilled occupational and physical therapy increases sensory perception, tolerance, and interpretation, develops improved coordination of movement, and teaches adaptations that magnify useful sensory input.

Sensory seeking and sensory sensitivity

Sensory seeking is seen in a child that intentionally crashes into the couch instead of sitting down, stomps or runs at every opportunity, and eagerly tears or crushes any paper. Receiving less sensory information from their muscles and joints often compels kids to seek out sensory input from movement, touch, sound, and even visual sources. The child rarely can explain why they act this way, or what it does for them. They know that they feel happier, more focused, or calmer after doing these actions. This can play havoc plans to have a child sit on a potty seat and become familiar with this new way of eliminating. They want to get up and run, shred the toilet paper, or play in the sink. For many kids new to potty training, sitting on the potty is utterly dull and meaningless. Addressing sensory seeking behavior before beginning toilet training will make for less work and fewer tears.

Tiffany wondered how James would ever manage to use the toilet by himself, considering how much the smells and sounds of pee and poop bothered him when she changed him in the bathroom during pre-training. He got upset if he couldn't flush the toilet immediately after he had a bowel movement, even before he was wiped. He would flush twice, but he absolutely had to flush his feces away and turn on the exhaust fan. But then the sound of the fan would bother him. It echoed inside the small bathroom in a way that really annoyed him. Tiffany tried to say as little as possible during diaper changes in the bathroom, because her voice would echo too.

The time when Jacqueline innocently left scented soap in the bathroom would be hard for everyone to forget. The soap was scented with cedar and pine. Tiffany's headache might begin to come back if she thought too much about how that smell hit her the first time she entered the powder room after the new soap was opened up. Not the smell of the soap. The smell of vomit after her son went into the powder room to wash his action figure off. James didn't cry when he went into the powder room. He just threw up his pizza from lunch. On her shoes. Her new shoes. The shoes that went right in the trash after she got her son cleaned up.

Sensory sensitivity can occur even when a child doesn't register and process sensory input effectively. Sensitivity to smells, sounds, lights, and being touched will detract from paying attention to elimination signals. It can also make a child resist going into the bathroom in the first place. They might want to be diapered *quickly to minimize sensations their find irritating or even distressing. Tiffany wondered how James would ever manage to use the toilet by himself, considering how much the smells and sounds of pee and poop bothered him when she changed him in the bathroom during pre-training. He got upset if he couldn't flush the toilet immediately after he had a bowel movement. He couldn't wait to be wiped first. James would flush twice, but he absolutely <u>had</u> to flush his feces away and turn on the exhaust fan. But then the sound of the fan would bother him. It echoed inside the small bathroom in a way that really annoyed him. Tiffany tried to say as little as possible during diaper changes in the bathroom, because her voice would echo too.*

A child's poor sensory processing can be missed or misinterpreted when they have significant struggles with coordinating movement. The kids who have only mild hypotonia are sometimes considered the most difficult to train, and for the wrong reasons. Mildly hypotonic children with mild sensory processing deficits are too often seen as having *only* behavioral issues. A child could be tolerant and flexible in the presence of everyday sensory input, but not when brought to an unfamiliar place or when there are multiple sources of sensory input coming at them at the same time. Their coping strategies aren't sufficient to handle the amount of rapid and complex processing needed in these environments. Illnesses or the loss of a key support person are two common stressors that can reveal the true extent of a child's sensory processing struggles.

The significant impact of sensory processing on toilet training is often minimized or even ignored by many professionals. This could be hard to understand, until you remember the maxim "If the only tool you have is a hammer, everything you see is a nail." Lack of familiarity with sensory processing disorders in general makes it more difficult to see them in a child with low muscle tone. Another familiar reaction from teachers and psychologists is to immediately refer parents and caregivers to speak with the child's occupational therapist. They may not adapt their original potty training plan, thinking that the OT will magically eradicate sensory processing problems coming from a physical condition. The reality is far more complex: hypotonic kids are rarely "cured" of their sensory processing struggles that affect toilet training. Their sensory issues are managed well, rather than cured. When their parents and their treatment team understand how to incorporate sensory-based treatment into toilet training, everyone wins.

Social/emotional issues

Many children are encouraged to watch potty videos and look at picture books featuring characters learning to use the toilet. These stories tell children that using the potty makes them a "big boy or girl" and that this is a desirable thing. The parents in these books and videos smile when the child in the story flushes the toilet, and everyone does the "potty dance". This works well because typically developing children often want to be seen as more mature, and they relish an adult's praise. When they accomplish something, they are proud. They want others to acknowledge their new skills. The adults are proud of the children and of themselves. Parents send videos and texts to relatives, sometimes taking photos of their kids with a "thumbs-up" sign. Everyone eagerly anticipates more freedom with social events and less need to clean up accidents.

This isn't always the same reaction when toilet training hypotonic kids. Although rarely mentioned by doctors, therapists, or special educators, potential social/emotional consequences of low tone exist. They include the fact that children often experience a longer period of physical dependency that influences both their self-image and how adults respond to them. Another issue is their persistent daily frustration with accomplishing the many tasks that require motor and sensory control. The primary social and emotional issues that come up are delayed maturity, learned helplessness, and low frustration tolerance. Finally, hypotonic children may have difficulty understanding that they will be initially given assistance that gradually fades away and will be replaced by full responsibility for their body and its needs. They are so used to constant support that the idea that it ends never occurs to them!

Kids who have been dependent on adults for physical skills often get used to being assisted. They may learn to assume that assistance will be offered even before they need it. Not needing to ask for what they want or need, a child with low muscle tone can defer responsibility for safety awareness to the point at which they don't think about something as simple as a loose towel on the floor where they need to walk. Some kids are used to only being asked to do a very select number of physical tasks during their day. Their fatigue or their need for considerable assistance can result in caregivers performing actions they are able to accomplish because it speeds things up. This situation changes during toilet training. A child will be both expected to follow instructions, but also to gradually sense what they need and when they need it. If they aren't naturally seeking independence in other parts of their life, it could be a shock.

Long after a typically developing child is building a healthy sense of separation and individuation, a kid with low muscle tone is still dependent for basic needs. Spending all those additional years dependent for diapering makes it seem as if dependence is the norm. Being helped feels "right"; it feels normal. Independence doesn't. It is not uncommon for a child with low muscle tone not to be motivated to be seen as older or more independent. It can be scary. Being left alone in the bathroom without assistance can be more frightening than inspiring. These new expectations can be felt as a burden for a child that has never been encouraged to assume control over their body and their actions.

Some children have been participating in diapering and dressing, but when they drop things, an adult picks those items up. When they forget something, an adult fetches it. They may not mind this. And neither do their caregivers. This is an essential "meta-skill" for ADL's. Being allowed to ignore the quality of their performance for self-care skills and not held accountable for the results is fairly common for many young children with physical delays. It can be a surprise to the child when the script flips during toilet training. No child should ever be called "lazy" or even "unmotivated". Given encouragement and a supportive environment, very few children won't shift their attitude to "Yes, I can!"

Attention, learning, and communication differences in hypotonia

We know that hypotonic children have unique learning styles, because every child has a unique learning style. They are all amazing little people, with their own personalities and interests that influence what they attend to, what questions they ask, and how they retain information. When it comes to learning self-care skills, there are some common learning, communication, and behavioral challenges seen that will need to be understood and managed. They do not preclude toilet training.

Typically developing kids learn well with direct instruction and learn through incidental learning. A parent will demonstrate and describe: "Johnnie, this is how to brush your back teeth". When a grandparent tells their sibling: "Hon, let me pour you some juice. Wait; put your cup on the table first" and then pours the juice, the child watching from their highchair is learning about how to pour a drink without being told what to do. This is incidental learning. Imitating adult actions is another method of learning. When a toddler grabs a pen and scrapes the wrong end onto the paper in a horizontal stroke and says "Wook; I wytin'!" they are showing us that they were watching our actions, can name them, and are refining what they learned through practiced imitation.

Hypotonic toddlers are working so hard to walk or talk that they may not be paying much attention to other people's actions. They may not have the essential grasp or strength to imitate a skill on their own, and their caregivers might not draw their attention to their demonstration in the same ways that they respond to typically developing kids. They could miss the phase of development in which imitation and incidental learning occur.

Using only verbal instructions may not be the most effective way to teach a self-care skill to a child with motor and sensory processing issues. They must listen, think, and move at the same time. For some children, explaining general actions could be insufficient for learning. Repeating the rules may not clarify the difference between "right now" and "every time you use the toilet". It can be helpful to remember what strategies worked for a particular child while they were learning to walk or climb stairs. Sharing this information with professionals improves the speed of a child's learning curve.

One of the most frustrating challenges when teaching practical skills to children is finding a way to help them generalize skill use in a variety of locations. Kids often learn a skill gradually and in a specific location. They may be able to use toilet in their parent's larger bathroom successfully but struggle to use the small powder room at a grandparent's home, and <u>completely</u> refuse to use the toilet in the stall at school. True independence is being able to use any toilet in any environment without assistance. This is a high bar for many children, but it can be done. Assuming that it comes naturally to every child is a mistake.

How an adult's behavior impacts potty training

Every adult brings with them their beliefs about how to toilet train, their understanding of hypotonia, their level of frustration tolerance, and their cultural influences on childcare and discipline. Caregivers who are unwilling to let children struggle a bit or who don't know how to modify their expectations for training a hypotonic child may offer help for toileting when it is not needed. Adults who think a child is being "lazy" (a word I would like to eradicate!) will frequently not provide supporting equipment or assistance to the child. Independent toileting can get delayed because of the adult's issues, not the child's issues.

Some parents feel guilty, thinking that they caused their child's issues through prenatal or genetic means. Witnessing their child struggle forces them to accept the reality of the diagnosis and face their fears about the future. Toilet training is when children take over control of their body and learn a major self-help skill. Diapering is both essential and intimate. It can be a moment of connection with a child. Some caregivers find that being needed in such an important way delays the moment when they must come to terms with the fact that their child is truly growing up. Seeing their "baby" become more independent, but struggle to do so, can be hard on them. They may find reasons not to move forward with toilet training.

Tiffany had known James's development was delayed almost from the start. He never got the hang of nursing; she switched to bottles and formula after the pediatrician became worried about his failure to gain weight at 6 weeks of age. She and her husband accepted the developmental pediatrician's diagnosis of idiopathic hypotonia and sensory processing disorder.
Tiffany wondered to this day if she had done anything to cause James's struggles.

33

She had pushed herself to work through morning sickness and increasingly high blood pressure. Or perhaps it was something in Corey's blood line. He had a cousin living in a group home who rocked while sitting in a chair at their holiday gatherings, and one of Corey's brothers had more than a passing resemblance to the character "Sheldon Cooper" on TV. On a bad night, these thoughts kept her up for hours.

Sometimes adults see their job as keeping a child happy because this child has so many other significant challenges. And this also brings up the fact that toilet training is…work. A lot of work. Crying or protesting children are almost always more work than calm and quiet kids. Paid caregivers might fear that they could lose their job if the children in their care are visibly unhappy or do not appear to like them. Adults could give in and take over all diapering or wiping so that a child will not resent them for being asked to fully participate. Finally, both parents and caregivers can be very short on time or have other pressing priorities. It seems faster in the short run to do more of the work or toileting rather than allow a child the time to practice and build skills. Many kids don't understand an adult's strong or conflicting emotions. An adult that is naturally bubbly but becomes angry or resentful can be confusing or even frightening for a child. A caregiver that makes a big fuss about success can trigger feelings of anxiety. These are the kids who won't enjoy "potty dance" celebrations. These risk-averse kids are worried that they will fail in the future and disappoint an adult. It is always difficult to explain to a caregiver or a partner that their well-meaning responses make the situation worse. Having to choose a response that helps a child feel safe and organized might feel constraining or make the adult feel they are being rejected as a person. This won't support a positive relationship with the hypotonic child.

Toilet training success requires that both parents and children switch their perspectives to a "can-do" attitude and start to imagine toileting independence as a reality.

It's time to make a plan.

Will symptom severity or age affect potty training?

This is a question that too many parents are hesitant to ask a healthcare provider or educator. Some parents are afraid that the answer will depress them or anger them. Others are certain that they know what the professional will say, so they don't bother to ask. Even more are swayed by any information on social media. One post will inspire them. The next will depress them. Inexperienced professionals may not be able to give them a clear answer.
Fearful or overwhelmed parents of kids with profound delays or dangerous behaviors have no energy left to ask this question. And then there are parents who believe that once their child develops better motor control, communication, and social/emotional skills, their self-care independence will come in naturally, like the first breezes of spring.

The correct response to this question is usually to ask more questions:

- *What additional diagnoses does a child have?*

- *Are any of these diagnoses progressive/degenerative?*

- *Has the child achieved many or most of the training readiness skills?*

- *If not, is there reason to believe they will <u>not</u> achieve those skills in the future?*

- *Do they have sufficient support at home and at school for training?*

Slow progression to full independence is not the same as a training failure. Many kids are trained for <u>daytime</u> urinary continence (the ability to control elimination) before the age of 5. They take much longer to use the toilet for bowel movements, and longer still to stay dry at night.

35

There *are* children that do not become completely independent in using the toilet in every setting, which includes using the toilet while out in public. They may be very inconsistent in their ability to sense urgency to pee or poop, or they need to use the bathrooms that are familiar for them to be successful. These kids tend to have delays in multiple areas of development. Their receptive language skills are below an 18-month level, and they often have problems with balance and coordination due to low muscle tone or spasticity. These children may also have a seizure disorder. They wear protective undergarments in some situations or perhaps in all situations, but often can use the toilet with adult assistance or just by following a familiar daily routine. Wearing a protective garment is an insurance policy for them against the disruption and possible agitation produced by toileting accidents.

Most hypotonic children will eventually become independent in using the toilet. Some children are trained early and quickly, with no more difficulty than their siblings. This book provides families and professionals with tools that can make toilet training faster as well as more successful!

Chapter 2

Readiness for Toilet Training: What Really Matters

Families decide to start toilet training for three primary reasons: outside events create pressure on them to begin training, they believe their child has achieved one or more of the critical potty training skills, or they have been told by a professional that it is time to do toilet training.

An outside event either requires the child to be toilet trained or makes being potty trained the logical choice. An example would be enrolling a child in a school or an activity that doesn't provide staff to change diapers. The alternative to training this child is for an adult to remain present at the school or available throughout the day to change a child's diaper. Another example of an event that makes it necessary for a family to want to toilet train would be the impending birth of a sibling. Parents who want to train their older child are hoping that they can avoid having *two* children in diapers. They expect (probably correctly!) to have much less time and attention for potty training after the new baby arrives. In another situation, a younger sibling might be ready for training. The family thinks they should try to train both kids at the same time. The second reason families decide to begin toilet training is when their child achieves a skill that parents or professionals believe is a precursor to successful training. It could be a language skill, a sign for elimination urgency, or a couple of dry diapers when they check on them first thing in the morning. Another skill that triggers parents to consider training is the child's ability to remove diapers and clothing. This isn't always a welcome sign; seeing a naked and soiled child running through the house, leaving a trail of wet or soiled clothing and diapers, can propel even the most hesitant parent to start potty training.

Tiffany, and her husband Corey, wondered if it was the right time to train James. Their toddler, Olivia, was getting so big. She was already recognizing the words for pee and poop, and she often got her own diaper when she needed a change! It seemed like perhaps they could train her at the same time as James. He did recognize the names of some foods and toys. During diaper changes he mostly tried to get out of the grasp of the unlucky adult that needed to change him. Tiffany thought that perhaps training them together would save time and give James both a buddy in training and a good model.

Tiffany's mom, Jacqueline, was their babysitter. Jacqueline was efficient, and she prided herself in how well she cared for James. Her definition of "cared for" was to do everything for him. She didn't want to teach him how to use a spoon; Jacqueline thought he would get too messy. She didn't want more work, and she prided herself on how nice he looked when they went out. Tiffany and Corey weren't certain she would be any more of an ally in potty training than she was for self-feeding. Corey secretly expected to see physical sparks fly when Jacqueline was told they were starting potty training.

The final reason to train is when the staff at school or a pediatrician recommends that a child start potty training. Their opinions and observations may be convincing enough that the child's family agrees that it is time to take the plunge. Sometimes a fresh pair of eyes and ears makes all the difference. A new teacher, a new therapist, or a consultant might be the person that sees opportunity and ability more clearly.

Deciding that it is time to train is different from knowing that the child and their family or other caregivers are ready to do toilet training. There are eight different types of readiness to consider. Not all readiness skills can be taught or purchased. Physical readiness is an example. This is why we do not train 6 month-old children to crawl up and sit, strapped in, on a tiny toilet. Even with targeted pre-training, the right physical skills, and talented/motivated caregivers, it is still possible for a child and their family to struggle with toilet training. In this chapter we will explore what true readiness looks like, and how to know if the time is right to do potty training. But first, it is important to understand that a child that isn't ready for toilet training is always ready for pre-training! Parents who consistently use targeted pre-training strategies before formal training see faster toilet training progress once a child is ready. They and their child have fewer surprises. There is less guesswork. Life is easier, regardless of the severity of a child's issues.

There <u>is</u> a wrong time for potty training

One of the most frustrating effects of failed toilet training is the realization that it was started for the right reasons, with the right attitude, but at the wrong time. There are many circumstances that make potty training a lot harder and more prone to failure. It is important for parents and caregivers to know what can trip up a terrific plan, when to pause training, and why pausing training without very good reasons can create downsides that make future attempts more difficult.

Starting toilet training during or immediately following a major change in the child's life is not recommended. This produces additional learning challenges while they are already experiencing stress. These include adding or subtracting a caregiver, adding a new sibling to the family, and big changes in the child's home or school. While their parents might be thrilled with their new kitchen/ great room combo, a child could need time to learn how to navigate this space. Changing the people in a child's daily life is equally disruptive. A new babysitter who says they are willing to do toilet training makes some parents feel like they won the lottery! Kids usually need some time to learn about their babysitter. Their babysitter is unlikely to understand the consequences of hypotonia and how to respond and react effectively. Think of timing toilet training as an airplane on a runway. Passengers need to be prepared to take flight.

Sean and Luke had already tried to train Bella in the past. Twice. It had not gone well. And by "not gone well", Sean meant "It was a disaster! It set her way back. Trying to train Bella also made my relationship with Luke temporarily rocky, just when we most needed to be a team." Thinking about the first time they tried, Sean and Luke now admit they no idea what they were doing. They bought the potty training book with the most star reviews, and started with very high hopes. Bella's screams and the poop that ended up on her, in her bed, on the floors, and on the walls, rapidly dashed those early hopes. The second time they tried, they hired a toilet training consultant to come to their home and do the a 'boot camp" approach. The trainer admitted that she didn't know that much about special needs toilet training, but she was game to try. She gave them a discounted rate for the extra 3 days she thought Bella would need.
There <u>was</u> some progress with the consultant. Bella was able to comprehend that

she would get 3 Cheez-Its for peeing in the toilet. It didn't seem clear to her that peeing on the floor or anywhere else was a problem. Things got very messy, and progress stalled. The consultant said she would return in a year, and of course, charge them again for her services.

What does true toilet training readiness look like?

There are many types of training readiness needed for success. Three of them are not "child" readiness; they are determined by whether the family or the school is ready to train. It is possible to begin training the child who lacks full readiness. Skills can be improved and enhanced as training goes along. A simple rule is that the greater difficulty the child has with learning complex skills, the more important it is that they have most of these readiness skills in place for formal training. Many families and professionals are surprised to learn that the level of skill needed to begin formal training might be lower than they expected.

1. **Financial:** Parents laugh about the luxury vacations they will be able to afford once they don't have to buy diapers or Pull-Ups. The truth is that there are also costs involved in toilet training. Ignoring the need to cover these costs leaves parents open to feeling hoodwinked, burdened, or flat-out short of funds in the middle of training. Feeling badly about not anticipating the financial costs of potty training weighs parents down just at the time when feeling confident would be incredibly useful.
    Disposable training pants and wipes aren't cheap. Reusable training pants and washcloths need to be purchased in quantity and then repeatedly laundered. Hypotonic children often use more wipes or toilet paper after peeing or pooping than most adults anticipate. This is often because they can struggle with motor coordination and compensate with needing more materials to wipe. It can also be because they drop materials or destroy them in some way that requires them to grab more. Accidents are expected and can be frequent during formal training; this means more loads of laundry every week. Some soiled underwear, and even some soiled clothing or (oops!) carpets and furniture, won't be salvaged after soiling. They will have to be replaced. All of this costs money as well as time.

Kids learn to manage their clothing more quickly if they have soft, loose clothing without complicated fasteners. This may mean that children need replacements to their wardrobe. Finally, equipment for potty training must be sourced. Most hypotonic kids will be able to use commercially available potty seats, footstools, or toilet inserts. These cost money or need to be borrowed if they aren't present in the home. There might be a potty seat that an older sibling used just a few years ago in the basement or garage. Kids with low muscle tone tend to train later than neurotypical children. This usually means they are larger in size. They may not fit on a potty seat made for a typically developing toddler. Even if they can fit on a seat, the equipment left over from a sibling could be the wrong choice for THIS child. It may be too wobbly, too distracting, or in some other way be a bad match. Using the wrong equipment can increase fear and resistance. This will require their family to borrow or buy the correct equipment for training.

Jordan and Lewis shared parenting as a part of their divorce agreement. They shared the expenses of parenting as well. Jordan's job as a member of the defense counsel for a multi-national company was intense, but it also meant that she had a good income. In her mind, it evaporated way too quickly every month. She could not believe how expensive private therapies were, but they were making a huge difference for Henry.

Her salary also paid for Danielle, her live-out nanny. Danielle was amazing. Jordan could not survive without her. Toilet training would eventually eliminate ordering the huge boxes of diapers and wipes that sat in the garage. Those savings were already spent: therapeutic swimming lessons were scheduled for the fall. The online parenting groups had convinced Jordan that swimming could help Henry stop tripping and start talking.

Is the family financially ready for toilet training?

- *Is there room in the family budget for disposable or cloth training pants, wipes, and/or washcloths?*
- *Can clothing for training be purchased, borrowed, or made?*

- *Is there room in the budget for extra laundry?*
- *Can potty seats, toilet inserts, footstools, etc. be purchased or borrowed?*

2. **Physiological:** Children's bodies need to have sufficient neurological maturation for continence to be ready for formal toilet training. "Continence" is the medical term for the ability to control emptying the bowel and the bladder. Most typically developing children reach this stage of physiological development to achieve daytime urinary continence by 18 to 24 months of age. Daytime control of bowels emerges slightly later. That doesn't mean that every child will have the other readiness skills at this age. The nerve pathways for active control of the external rectal sphincter muscle needs to be fully developed for bowel continence. Children also need to have consistent formed bowel movements. This means that their feces are solid enough and they do not switch constantly between diarrhea and constipation. Kids with hypotonia may not pee or poop as consistently as a neurotypical child, but their elimination pattern needs to be reasonably predictable. They cannot be leaking feces or urine throughout the day. Diet, active movement, and digestive health all contribute to regulating intestinal activity. Medications, nutritional supplements, and gut disorders can have direct or indirect impacts on a child's ability to have predictable and formed bowel movements. It may be necessary to address digestive issues before formal toilet training begins.

Without the ability of the urinary sphincter muscles to be under conscious control, retaining urine until it can be released voluntarily, a child will not be able to achieve continence. A child who can focus awareness on sensory cues and daily routines may be continent during the day without fully established neurological maturation of these muscles. That changes for nighttime. Refined neurological control of urinary sphincter muscles and neurohormonal control of nighttime urination are essential for complete continence. Neurophysical development for nighttime control can take longer than for daytime control. It is common for neurotypical children under the age of 6 to occasionally wet their bed at night and still be considered completely normal. The bladder is a hollow organ lined with smooth muscle fibers, and it must grow large enough and strong enough to hold some urine during the day and more throughout the night. This is achieved without a child's active control. It is not the same as the ability to "hold it", like your mom told you to do while on a long car ride!

Most child development experts consider the ability to keep a diaper dry for 1.5-2 hours during the day during the day a good indicator of adequate physical maturation for daytime urinary continence. Adults should start checking a child's diapers every 10-15 minutes when they can monitor continence over the space of a few hours. By keeping track of a child's natural elimination routines, a distinct pattern should emerge as the child develops the physiological readiness for toilet training. Even if a child is only dry for 45 minutes at first, adults will be recording those dry periods and looking for a gradual increase in length of time with a dry diaper to assess adequate physiological readiness for toilet training.
A child needs to be able to sit on a potty seat or toilet with enough stability to both <u>be</u> safe and <u>feel</u> safe. It is very difficult for a child to relax enough to allow elimination when they think that they could fall. If a child seems uncomfortable, even though they look stable, they may need more time to become confident or need different equipment. A child should be able to walk (or crawl very quickly) to the potty independently to be ready for formal training. Frequent accidents frustrate and discourage children. No one fails to use a diaper successfully. Kids figure that out amazingly quickly and become resistant to potty training.

Sean and Luke watched Bella navigate the playground climbing structure while both dads held their respective breaths. She was fearless. That wasn't a positive. Bella insisted on climbing to the highest part of anything if she could, and it was anyone's guess whether she would jump or fall. At 8, she was getting big to catch. Even for Sean, who was 6'4". His back wasn't getting any younger, and she wasn't getting any safer. This didn't mean that she didn't slide off their kitchen chairs while still holding her hamburger. She could climb like a cat, but not consistently stay sitting on a chair...

Finally, kids with low muscle tone need to have adequate sensory processing for training. Being able to sense and interpret urgency signals in time to get to the toilet is essential. Sensing their posture as they sit or stand, and sensing clothing placement are two specific ways sensory processing skills that contribute to toileting success. Knowing that their underwear isn't pushed down far enough over their buttocks without seeing their clothing, and adjusting it in time, might make all the difference between soiling clothing and not soiling. It doesn't end there. The sensations of elimination can be intense, even overwhelming for some children. The environment of the bathroom can be equally difficult to handle. Combining them together may derail a child who has never struggled with being diapered in their bedroom once. It isn't about ignoring the sensory stimulation; it is about processing it smoothly and quickly enough to use the toilet and go on with their day.

Is a child physiologically ready for toilet training?

- *Does the child wake up in the morning or from a nap with a dry diaper at least 3-4x/week?*
- *Is their diaper dry for at least 1.5-2 hours while awake?*
- *Are their bowel movements formed and pain-free?*
- *Can the child sit on a potty seat or toilet seat safely and independently without fear?*
- *Can the child tolerate the sounds of a toilet flushing, water flowing, fans running, and people speaking in the bathroom?*
- *Can the child remain calm and attentive while being diapered and dressed?*
- *Can they sense their posture and clothing placement sufficiently for safe toileting?*

3. **Communication Readiness:** Children need to have basic language skills for toileting. It doesn't have to be verbal communication. A child who can communicate about toileting effectively using signs or pictures is capable of being toilet trained. Their receptive language skills (understanding words/signs/graphics) do not need to be greater than an 18-month level for success. A child's speech therapist or teacher can help determine if using signs or pictures would be <u>more</u> effective or less effective than

verbal language. The child who has some verbal language may be more functional using signs or PECS for potty training. This is because a task that requires effective communication as quickly as possible (pee doesn't wait for anyone!) requires using the most efficient communication strategy. It is important to recognize that using pictures or signs in toilet training while developing verbal communication skills is NOT a sign of failure and is not necessarily a risk for progress in building verbal skills.

Does a child have the communication skills for toilet training?

- *Does the child recognize their name when called?*
- *Can the child follow a simple __familiar__ instruction with only a brief verbal prompt or gesture? Example: An adult says, "Up, pull pants UP!" while tapping the waistband of a child's shorts. The child reaches for the waistband and wiggles it up an inch.*
- *Does the child communicate that they need a diaper change? Examples are bringing an adult a clean diaper, bringing the adult to the changing table, or pointing to their diaper before __or__ after they pee or poop.*
- *Does the child understand words/signs/graphics for body parts and simple physical actions? Non-verbal indications of comprehension would be touching the front of her diaper when asked if it is "wet" or standing up when an adult signs "Stand".*

4. **Cognitive Readiness:** Like communication, the cognitive skills needed for toilet training readiness are at approximately the 18-month level of intelligence. Of course, many children with low muscle tone have cognitive skills that far exceed this level but their motor skills are lower. Their greater comprehension, memory and problem solving will help them make faster gains. A child needs to recall simple routines and to understand why they are being praised or rewarded. Without this, kids have no idea why they are taken to the potty or why they get a treat. Some children don't respond consistently to verbal praise or physical affection, but they understand why they got an immediate treat.
Parents of children with complex developmental delays such as Down syndrome and Prader-Willi syndrome may have been encouraged to wait

until a child's cognitive abilities are more advanced, sometimes waiting well after the age of 4 or 5. At this age, the decision may be to begin pre-training. One risk of waiting so long is simple: after years of diapering, children can assume that their parents WANT them to use a diaper.

Is a child cognitively ready for toilet training?

- *Can the child recall 2-3 steps to open a container or assemble a toy, even if they need physical assistance to accomplish it?*
- *Can a child recognize that the received a reward or praise because of their action?*
- *Can the child remember and anticipate simple daily routines at home or school?*

5. **Social/Emotional Readiness:** Kids need to be able to stay calm and cooperate while learning a complex but frustrating new skill; a skill that may not make any sense to them at first. Wanting to please an adult isn't necessary for training, but it does make it much easier. The Baby Whisperer, a.k.a. Tracy Hogg, said that the easiest time to train a child is when they have achieved the ability to stand and manage clothing, can understand and recall routines, but still remain more motivated by adult praise and interaction than by being defiant and controlling adults. Anyone that has tried to train an older child knows <u>exactly</u> what she is talking about. Children with low muscle tone that have been discouraged or feel over-controlled can have difficulty reacting appropriately to praise. A child may need a particular word to be used when they are praised. Something that is meaningful and motivating to them.

Children often want to be off exploring independently. Sitting on the toilet feels like being trapped. They need to be willing to sit still on the potty for short periods to become physiologically comfortable and physically relax enough to pee and poop. Some kids with limited sensory registration need to sit quietly long enough to sense whether they are ready to "go". They can't sense it while "on the run". The ability to remain sitting on request, even when they do not understand the rationale <u>and</u> they have other things they would prefer to do, is important for successful formal training. A child should have some motivation to be independent with other daily living skills before beginning toilet training. This includes wanting to finger feed and taking the initiative to remove socks and hats.

Toilet training in middle and later toddlerhood can be much harder than in the early toddler years; defiance and even withholding become more appealing than receiving a small treat. This response is normal social and emotional development for older toddlers. That doesn't make it easy to handle! It is very frustrating to realize that a once-sweet child has now eagerly drawn a line in the sand and dared the adult to cross it! Managing defiance and withholding as behavior issues are covered later in this book. Children also need the ability to endure the experience of accidents without becoming overly frustrated or feel shame. They may feel embarrassment or fear. These reactions could trigger a child's refusal to use the toilet. Older children desire privacy even as they need adult assistance. Because of their emotional immaturity, they may not know that this is happening. What they do sense it that being toilet trained doesn't feel good but neither does having a diaper. They are like out-of-sorts teens who don't know why there are unhappy and make everyone "pay" for it!

Corey and Tiffany wondered if James would ever do what they told him to do without a scene. Granted, he was only 3. But their toddler Olivia turned around and smiled if you called her name. She also smiled broadly if you mentioned the words "snack", "outside", or "doggie". She did have her out-of-control moments, but Olivia could be calmed down in half the time it took to settle James. His fits were legendary. You needed to be in protective gear when you tried to take something away from him, or if you didn't give him what he wanted quickly enough. Both of his parents felt powerless at times.

Is a child socially and emotionally ready for potty training?

- *Can a child respond positively to praise or rewards?*
- *Is the child showing interest in independence in other self-care skills?*
- *Is the child interested in wearing underwear?*
- *Can a child wait briefly (at least 30 seconds) for a requested drink or toy?*

- *Does the child cooperate with simple requests more frequently than they become defiant?*
- *When a child spills food or breaks a toy, are they easily consoled and willing to try eating or playing again?*

6. **Clothing Management:** If a child stands there like a store mannequin while being dressed, then they need to level up their dressing skills for toilet training. Children being trained should at least be able to assist an adult with getting their pants up or down. They may not be fast or effective yet, but they need to be able to be actively involved in clothing management. Children who stand in front of the toilet playing with their superhero toy while their mother positions them to urinate aren't learning much about independent toileting.

The limitations in proprioception and kinesthesia from hypotonia routinely make it harder for kids to rapidly recognize elimination urgency. This is knowing that you need to use the potty…right now! Once the signal is processed, they don't have a lot of time to act to avoid an accident. Kids who cannot manage their own clothing are much more likely to have an accident. Adults aren't always able to get to them in time. Discouragement and embarrassment from accidents is a huge reason for children to refuse to continue training. Being able to manage clothing could make all the difference for a child with low muscle tone.

Luke loved dressing Bella in the cutest outfits. She was his own personal Barbie doll; the one he was never allowed to have as a young gay boy. He and his husband Sean had paid a surrogate to carry her, and she was his heart. Full stop. Sean knew this and he loved that Luke was absolutely over the moon about their daughter. But she wasn't so little anymore. She was 8. Being non-verbal and not toilet trained meant that all those layers of fabric from his mother-in-law's frilly clothes she bought Bella were a daily physical challenge even for diapering. Bella was no help at all. She spent most of her time fighting to get off the changing table. She could bite him if he took too long. She had a few adult teeth now. Some days it was like wrestling with a cute little…alligator.

Is a child ready to deal with clothing management?

- *Can the child assist in any way with clothing during their diaper change?*
- *Can the child take off their pajamas or an unfastened coat?*
- *Will the child start to pull off their clothes to get into the bathtub?*
- *Has the child pulled off their hat and socks independently?*

1. **Time and Attention:** Regardless of whether gradual training or intensive training is the plan, the adults doing potty training will need considerable time and attention for it to be successful. If the plan is to do "boot camp" training, the primary adult doing training will be focusing on the child to the point that many of their daily responsibilities will need to be shouldered by someone else in the household. This is even harder when a hypotonic child has siblings. They have needs and deserve attention too. It becomes harder still if the child training is a twin whose sibling is at a different phase in training. For nighttime training, a parent needs to get up during the night to bring a sleepy (and usually wobbly) child to the potty or change their wet sheets if they didn't make it in time.
Even the use of the gradual approach to toilet training has adults spending time focusing attention on a child's elimination routines to learn when they are most likely to pee and poop. Parents will be adjusting a child's diet to ensure that there is enough fiber and hydration throughout the day. Doing laundry and cleaning up accidents takes time out of an already busy day. Being consistent with focused attention and coming up with creative ways to stick with the plan demands time, attention, and determination. Parents who aren't ready for this are in for some big surprises. Inconsistent delivery of formal toilet training might be the primary reason for failure. It could have little to do with a child's muscle tone or other skills.

Kids with low muscle tone are often in therapies when they aren't in school. They have full days. Days that don't leave a lot of time to sit on the potty. Some parents choose to have the school staff do toilet training just because of this issue. Others decide that they can carve out time for a "boot camp" more easily than spending time every day slowly making

49

progress. Both approaches to toilet training require time, and many hypotonic kids do both. They do one or more "boot camps" to jump start progress, and they need gradual focus to refine skills.

Jordan and her ex, Lewis, felt they already had their hands full, and full all of the time. They divorced almost immediately after Henry was born. Lewis's mom, Sharon, was a retired special education teacher. Jordan thought that her ex mother-in-law would like to become Henry's de facto team leader. She also thought that Lewis didn't seem to have a problem with that idea. To her, it appeared that he thought that it would give him a free pass on the hard decisions they had to make. Sharon had already told her son that she was an expert in potty training. "Some expert!", thought Mia. "She taught in a regular preschool for 10 years, and she thinks she knows more about medications and neurology than our neurologist and pediatrician combined. At least in HER own mind." The truth was that Sharon was their son's caregiver after school every weekday but she would leave for Florida in the fall. If Henry wasn't potty trained by then, someone else would have to take over childcare. Who and how were the big questions.

Is there sufficient time and attention available for toilet training?

- *Who will monitor diapers and behavior to learn elimination frequency and timing?*
- *Who will focus on menus, diet, and digestion?*
- *Is a child's schedule flexible enough for a "potty intensive"?*
- *Who will do the training during a "potty intensive"?*
- *Who will take over other household responsibilities during intensive training?*
- *How will the rest of a child's team be updated on progress and concerns?*
- *For night training, who will do nighttime potty breaks and manage accidents?*

8. **Appropriate Equipment:** Selected the right equipment for toilet training gives a child the best chance at success. Even if their muscle tone is only mildly low, they deserve the optimal positioning for fast and easy prog-

ress. Unless a hypotonic child is very young, they won't fit on a toddler training potty. Even if they can sit on one, they are too close to the floor to get up safely with their pants around their ankles. The choices for toilets largely fall into three simple categories: regular toilets, toilet seat inserts, and stand-alone potties. Most smaller children use a toilet seat insert and a footstool or some other device that allows their feet to touch a stable surface while sitting or standing. Older kids are tall enough to sit on the toilet with their feet on the floor. While it is possible to find and install a preschool-sized toilet, it is usually only done if the child will have easy access to this bathroom most of the day, and there are other toilets for older children and adults in the home.

Finding the <u>perfect</u> piece of equipment may not be possible or necessary. Many kids do well with all three types of toilet set-ups. The larger the number of challenges a child has, the more important it will be to get exactly the right item. Sometimes the right thing to do is to get rid of things in the bathroom, not add more. Bathrooms have tile floors, and many families use small rugs around or near the toilet. Loose rugs become both accidentally soiled and act as tripping hazards during toilet training.

There are other toileting items to consider, such as whether a child needs permanent or temporary grab bars. Larger wipes and thicker toilet paper are additional items that can make toileting easier and safer.

Is the appropriate equipment for training available?

- *Does the available equipment fit the child?*
- *Is the equipment sturdy and stable for sitting and standing?*
- *Can the child place their feet flat on a footstool or on the floor while sitting or standing at the sink to wash their hands?*
- *Can the child get on and off the toilet independently or with supervision?*
- *Have bathroom hazards and distractions been removed?*

Doing a complete readiness assessment allows a child's whole team to focus attention and prepare for success. If a child isn't ready, or if the team isn't ready, they now have more of a sense of what to do. They know which skills are necessary to begin training, and which are not essential. If pre-training is the right choice, everyone moves forward knowing this is the plan.

Chapter 3

How Diet, Digestion, and Medications Impact Toilet Training

It can be incredibly difficult to successfully toilet train a child that has unpredictable or uncomfortable urination and bowel movements. It will be hard to know when to bring them to the potty, and if a new strategy or schedule has helped them or not. Both the child and the adults doing training become frustrated and discouraged. A child's diet, their medications, and digestive problems can absolutely derail the best toilet training plan.

Henry was predictably unpredictable; he was always all over the place when it came to knowing when he would poop. It could be in the most inconvenient times, and multiple times a day. Then not poop for a few days, which made his mom so anxious that she could become constipated as well! In truth, she had her issues with food and digestion as well. Always a picky eater as a kid, Jordan had a short time in college where she was anorexic. She still became anxious when she ate anywhere else but at home. Henry's picky eating and digestive issues triggered her anxieties more than anyone knew; she didn't even tell her therapist how she felt. She didn't want to fully admit how rough things got sometimes. And he certainly picked up on her issues. No language, lots of stimming, but that kid picked up on her food preferences and her stress around food. She saw it.

An important cornerstone of effective early toilet training is knowing when a child is most likely to need to pee and poop. Without that information, taking them to the potty will always be a guessing game. A game in which "losing" means everyone loses <u>confidence and motivation,</u> and kids don't make the connection between sitting and elimination.

If a child has already emptied their bladder into their diaper, they can't pee into the toilet until more urine is produced by their kidneys. Motivation has nothing to do with it. It takes time for kidneys to work, and timing is everything in potty training. This goes double for bowel movements. Once a child has had a bowel movement, they can't have another until their intestines move feces into the rectum in enough quantity to trigger elimination. If you miss the "window", they may not poop again until the next day, or even the following day.

Elimination Communication (EC) theory has many critics, but EC has a very useful principle that makes potty training a hypotonic child easier: adults pay intensely focused attention to a child's signals that they are ready to "go potty". Most adults with childcare experience know some of the general signs: kids who hide behind the couch as they prepare to poop into their diaper, and children who hold their crotch or cross their legs as they pee into their diaper. Using EC-level focused attention during pre-training, adults become very good at identifying a hypotonic child's signals that they need to "go", without the child saying anything at first. Their lack of verbal communication or their difficulty requesting assistance will be less of a barrier to starting successful toilet training. As a child builds more skills, they need to sense and respond to their body's signals promptly. It starts with the adults around them noticing outward signs of urgency and communicating this to the child.

The science of digestion

As children get physiologically closer to training readiness, their natural elimination schedules become more predictable. They may have bowel movements 30-minutes or so after their meal(s). This is a physiological response, not a preference. A child could also routinely pass feces when waking up in the morning, or when waking from a nap. Again, the neurochemical and physical changes as we move from sleep into wakefulness contribute to this response. Bowel evacuation (a fancy medical word to describe feces leaving the rectum) is more complex than urination. Understanding an individual's patterns will matter as much as knowing the general physiological principles. As solid food enters the stomach, the stretching of the stomach (muscles again!) and the reflexive opening of the entrance of the small intestine will stimulate contraction of the small and large intestines. Rhythmic muscular contraction (peristalsis, for those who want the medical terms!) moves digested food in the direction of the rectum for evacuation. Emptying the rectum requires relaxation of the external rectal sphincter muscle and is supported by active contraction of abdominal muscles against the intestines, creating greater intra-abdominal pressure. There can be issues for hypotonic kids at every step along the path from the stomach to the anus. For most families, awareness and general support for digestion will be enough. For some children, a gastroenterologist's assistance is essential. But do not think that a GI specialist is a specialist in toilet training! They may admit it, but the truth is that even if they are parents, they have been working long hours most days while someone <u>else</u> was running the potty training plan.

Kids urinate about 30-45 minutes after a substantial drink that was taken when their stomach was empty. Our kidneys filter blood at a predictable pace unless we have a condition that affects this process. A very full bladder will empty by itself if intense pressure overrides conscious contraction of the external urinary sphincter muscle. Both urination and bowel movement frequency and transit time (speed) after a meal will be affected by the amount and the content of a child's meal. Urination could take slightly longer when food is consumed along with liquids, or when the liquid contains large amounts of fat or protein. A milkshake is a good example of this type of liquid. A meal that is low in fiber will take longer to digest, and food with a large amount of fat triggers faster passage through the intestine.

Parents and caregivers need to be aware of a child's unique elimination patterns to identify when problems occur and get them to the potty in time to avoid frustrating and discouraging accidents. This prevents aggravating a child that sits on the toilet for 15 minutes but only pees a tiny amount because they haven't had anything to drink for the past 2 hours. When children can connect the sensations of elimination urgency to the need to use the toilet, formal training is far faster and easier. It should start in targeted pre-training and build from there.

Why hypotonic kids have more digestive problems

The motor, sensory, and behavioral issues that affect kids with low muscle tone can make establishing and observing regular intake and elimination routines more challenging. A child with more severe challenges is very likely to develop complications that affect toilet training. The good news is that addressing these challenges makes a child healthier, happier, and moves them closer to being able to learn the skills of toilet training.

Hypotonic kids may take medications for other medical issues or to treat behavioral problems. The effect of some medications, or the effects of combining medications and supplements, can contribute to difficulties with healthy elimination patterns. Natural supplements have as much risk as pharmaceuticals. These effects include a decrease or increase in appetite, changes in gut motility, and altered food absorption. A child could have all three of these complications from a single medication or supplement. Or they might only happen when something is added to a child's prescription. The most common medications that contribute to constipation in children are reflux medications and anticonvulsants. Antibiotics and some types of reflux medications are the most common drugs that create diarrhea. These medications may be essential to a child's health and safety. They should <u>never</u> be discontinued without the prescriber's consent. Discussing any change in medication must be done with the guidance of a child's healthcare providers.

Pediatricians and pediatric gastroenterologists can help determine what is contributing to a child's elimination issues. They can also identify if there is an additional condition that requires medical treatment. These healthcare providers may need to be consulted before formal potty training begins to get the best results. The physical issues associated with hypotonia contribute to digestive problems. It is common for children with low muscle tone to have less frequent bowel movements than children with normal muscle tone. Low tone in the abdominal muscles produces less intra-abdominal pressure, and therefore less beneficial external intestinal stimulation. Children with low muscle tone frequently have lower overall levels of physical activity compared with their peers. They are more likely sitting or lying down for longer periods of the day, and when active, they sustain this for shorter periods. This reduces their ability to build muscle and stimulate intestinal motility.
The smooth muscles of the intestines that move food along toward elimination can become less efficient as well. They are significantly impacted by autonomic nervous system functioning. This system, in turn, is affected in its vitality and efficiency by emotional agitation, sleep disruptions, and sensory

processing problems.   Children with autonomic issues that affect digestion can have loose stool one day and constipation the rest of the week.

Constipation and diarrhea

Diarrhea and constipation cause more than belly aches.   These problems create sensory-based issues and emotional issues that can stop all progress in potty training.   Young children do not understand why they are in such discomfort, but they know exactly what they want to avoid: using the potty! They are not afraid of the <u>toilet</u> per se; they are afraid of being in pain and older children may be afraid of feeling embarrassed by soiling or receiving enemas.   They now associate these negative feelings with the potty.   This can be conscious, but it can also be an unconscious response that they deny when an adult asks a child about their thinking.   Young children cannot be expected to have mature insights.   Even if they want desperately to please, their anxiety around elimination problems will make it difficult for them to relax and have a normal bowel movement.   Again, it is nearly impossible to successfully do formal toilet training when these issues exist.

James was in the middle of a very difficult bowel movement. Tiffany held him, massaging his belly. He hadn't pooped in about 4 days after she stopped giving him the daily mild laxative. She made that choice because he hated how it tasted. Somehow, he could detect it diluted or mixed into anything. But now she truly regretted her decision. There was nothing like one of her children suffering to make her want to cry too. Now she had to decide if she should give him an enema. James would need to be held down to administer it without harming him. Tiffany hated the idea of holding her son down, but she knew that if she brought him to pediatric urgent care, they would give him an enema there. No soft music, no cuddling, just bright lights and strangers. True, they were a little faster with the tubing, and they were nice enough to him. Being in a strange place with strange people in masks was harder for James. And all of this because she had dared to believe that they were making progress and could stop the laxative…

Some children with low muscle tone have small and loose bowel movements multiple times a day. This is often due to their diet or the medications that they are taking. Another common reason is chronic constipation. Loose feces are "slipping past" the impacted stool and leaking out. Sitting on the toilet increases the pain from the hard stool in their rectum, so they refuse to stay there. Chronic constipation can weaken their pelvic floor muscles. In a vicious cycle, weaker muscles cannot help a child empty their bowels and increase their constipation.

A child's menu can be either the problem or the solution

Narrowed food types and textures can contribute to both constipation and diarrhea. Kids with difficulty chewing and swallowing often prefer to eat soft foods with little fiber. Excessive amounts of carrots, squash, bananas, and dairy contribute to constipation. They may be unable to safely eat other foods, or they may be afraid to do so. Because fiber is one key to smooth, regular, and pain-free bowel movements in almost everyone, this causes issues for many kids. Fiber in a diet adds bulk to stool and stimulates digestive motility. *Lack of bulky stool diminishes the sensory signals that are essential to initiate the smooth muscle contractions needed for the intestines to move feces into the rectum.*

Very high fiber diets, on the other hand, can result in diarrhea. This is seen with children who eat large quantities of whole grain crackers and breads or eat large amounts of foods high in pectin. Diarrhea is common with food allergies or sensitivities, and excessive amounts of sugar are known to contribute to diarrhea. The parents and caregivers of kids that refuse to eat or drink for long periods will see that this refusal directly affects their digestive ease. Children that appear to be continent may not be making any progress in potty training at all; they simply don't consume enough to fill their bladder or rectum for long periods.

Every child reacts differently to single foods or combinations of foods. For every child that becomes constipated when they eat too many bananas, there will be a child that develops diarrhea after eating them. The most frequent dietary source of sugar in a child 's diet are large amounts of fruit juice. If a preferred juice turns out to be the problem, slowly watering down their juice will gradually decrease their sugar intake. A pediatric probiotic supplement may help regulate bowel function.

Tiffany decided to revisit the subject of the family meal. Once she learned that so many of James's fave foods were likely culprits in his constipation, she made some adjustments. Tiffany decided that for her first attempt, she would slowly blend in some whole-grain macaroni into his mac-and-cheese dinners. When she got to the 50/50 stage, she went for broke and did 75/25, without even a wince from him! There was a bonus; Corey and Olivia loved it as well. She had a new recipe that everyone would eat without an argument.

To add a wider range of nutrients and fiber to a child's diet, there are recipes that make small additions harder for a child to perceive. Recipe books and manufactured products using vegetable and bean purees can avoid arguments and tears. They use clever substitutions to adapt child-friendly recipes such as macaroni and cheese, chocolate chip cookies, and brownies. There are obvious pros and cons to this subterfuge. Adding new foods can risk sensitivities or allergies, so families should discuss this strategy with their treatment team. Be aware that extremely picky eaters may be able to detect a change in flavor and refuse these foods if the flavor or texture changes are significant. Gradually mixing in small amounts of a new food into a favorite recipe can successfully avoid triggering these "super-taster's" refusals.

Regardless of the reason for recent or chronic digestive issues, the pre-training period is the best time to come up with solutions for digestive distress or irregularity. Then families have to consider whether past constipation or reflux problems have left residual emotional scars and habits that will complicate potty training.

Old (solved) problems can create new toileting issues

Some children with low muscle tone had complex physical problems from birth that impacted feeding and digestion. There may have been early issues with latching onto the breast or poor bottle feeding. Their attention to eating and drinking may have been inconsistent or even aversive; they were not focused on copying the mature actions of others and enjoying the social components of mealtime. Reflux or allergic reactions frequently emerge in the first months or years of life. These can be difficult issues to solve. They often are emotionally

59

charged. A parent can feel that they are failing their child even though they logically know that they are doing everything they can. This is an emotional reaction. They can feel rejected by the child, and the child can react with fear to being fed. In fact, it is often emotionally easier for families and children to handle illnesses and injuries than to handle feeding problems.

It may have taken some time to get the right treatment for these problems. The fear, the frustration, and other emotions the family and the child experience will not be fully forgotten by anyone right away. Because young kids may still struggle with communication and do not have mature emotional reactions or insight, they cannot tell adults that they remember those days and are afraid of throwing up or having a painful bowel movement. What is seen instead is an increase in aversive or defiant behavior or a general sense of avoidance or agitation when pre-training increases the focus on elimination. When they refuse to drink larger amounts of fluid or become upset when constantly offered fluids during "boot camp", it could be bad memories resurfacing instead of reactions to current events.

Using positive mealtime routines for successful potty training

Predictable mealtime routines are helpful for almost every child during pre-training and during formal toilet training. Meals served at a regular time, in a set location, have a very important role. They help a child prepare for a similar new routine: eliminating in one location. Kids who are non-verbal benefit even more from this change because they are more dependent on environmental cues to learn and perform tasks. This change might be very different from the usual mealtime experience. A child may have been roaming around the house holding food, eating in front of a screen, or repeatedly returning to the dining table to be fed a bite or two. It could take time to help them alter their mealtime habits. This is a great goal for targeted pre-training, even though it isn't a specific toileting skill.

Regular mealtimes make digestion, and therefore elimination, more predictable. Inconsistent mealtimes and constant grazing have the opposite effect. It is nearly impossible to monitor intake for a child who grazes or sips from a cup throughout the day. Offering more regular mealtimes doesn't mean adults decrease the amount of food or drink provided. If anything, children who don't graze or sip through the day are often hungrier and thirstier during meals. They can consume more food and drink. They could also be more open to eating healthier foods. Because kids consume more food and drink at a single time, they receive greater sensory stimulation from a fuller belly and bladder. When a child connects this sense of fullness and knows it is elimination urgency: they need to pee or poop!

There are additional benefits to routine mealtimes that aren't related to toilet training; children who sit for a meal are learning more about social interaction, including patience and following directions. The social and communication opportunities that happen when eating with others directly benefit toilet training. Other members of the family and paid caregivers will change their perception of a sibling who is now able to participate in family meals. When kids are treated more like other members of the family at the dinner table, it changes everyone for the better.

Jordan noticed that Angela, her 10-year-old, was talking to Henry more these days. "What changed?" she asked herself. It came to her during dinner. Henry was now sitting for at least 5-7 minutes at the beginning of every family meal. He didn't say much, but he was smiling and laughing more. He could pass a roll or a napkin to his sister. She was responding. Angela started talking to him like a big sister instead of always ignoring him. Jordan decided that they had waited too long to make this change.

The search for a support team

A good team of professionals can make all the difference in addressing the digestive issues that complicate toilet training a hypotonic child. A child's pediatrician is an important member of every team. Families must offer them as much information as possible about a child's toilet training challenges. More information helps them diagnose problems and recommend possible medical solutions. They may make referrals rather than address issues directly. Parents need to share any side effects of medications that are impacting eating and elimination. Any nutritional supplements or alternative medicines should be reported. Due to the tight schedules in most medical practices, most parents need a game plan to get the best results. Preparing a solid history of digestive issues, focusing on one or two primary concerns, and focusing on the issues that a provider's training is most likely to address will work better than arriving without any preparation at all.

Finding new or additional medical professionals could be helpful if a problem has been persistent or is getting worse. Motility specialists are gastroenterologists with additional training in treating constipation and diarrhea. A registered dietician can help select foods and design healthy meals and snacks that will support smooth elimination. A feeding therapist (usually a speech or occupational therapist with specialized training) could be essential to address a child's difficulties swallowing, biting, or chewing. These providers have experience with hypotonic kids and offer practical strategies to use at home. Early Intervention programs often provide these services without charge. Private insurance may cover the charge for these services when they are prescribed by a physician.

Jordan decided it was time to get some advice from a nutritionist that specialized in ASD. This time she would come clean about her eating issues too. The nutritionist assured her that she would not disclose that information to Lewis. The first meeting with the nutritionist went well. He suggested that Jordan consider some new ideas. She would keep a record of how much he was eating and drinking after she stopped letting him graze all day and sip non-stop from a sippy cup. It became obvious that he was indeed pooping about 30-40 minutes after breakfast, as long as it was a big enough breakfast.

Henry was also a champ at soaking a diaper in about the same amount of time. Give him a box of chocolate milk, and you could set your watch for him to pee. The nutritionist told her that temporarily increasing Henry's sugar consumption wasn't a guarantee of a crazy day, but it could give him diarrhea. He showed her the scientific studies that supported this claim. Jordan had to admit there had been plenty of birthday cakes that didn't seem to make him act up, and lots of other times where he ate a slider with fries and had to leave an event shortly after.

Chapter 4

The Basics of Pre-Training Magic

Parents and professionals can be actively building a child's toilet training readiness skills long before a child is old enough, stable enough, or motivated enough for formal training. It can start before a child can hold a toy with both hands. It can start before a child is able to speak. And it can start before a child is able to sit on a potty seat. Building readiness skills will be woven into the child's current daily routine without caregivers devoting considerable time or money to the process. This includes the tasks that they do every day: diapering, feeding, and playing with the hypotonic child. Building skills that matter for toilet training can enhance the emotional relationship between an adult and the child. The skills that develop will have beneficial effects on learning other important skills such as walking, talking, and dressing.

How? The magic of _targeted_ pre-training.

Parents, nannies, and babysitters aren't the only ones who do targeted pre-training. Teachers and therapists can also build a child's toileting readiness skills within their classroom or clinic space. It doesn't require ADL (activities of daily living) goals on an IFSP or IEP. Parents, teachers, and therapists will be surprised and relieved to know that they probably have been doing a few of these pre-training techniques already; they just haven't recognized them as important parts of toilet training readiness! This chapter reviews three pre-training techniques used to build many of the readiness skills in chapter 2; they are Potty Talk, Potty Models, and Potty Play. It goes on to describe the specific technique that turns a regular diaper change into a teaching moment: *Collaborative Diapering.*

What about the kids who are years away from using the toilet?

Even if formal toilet training is clearly months or years in the future, it is possible to use targeted pre-training to move things in the right direction. It can be used even if the child's team is uncertain that a child will ever be fully independent in the bathroom. Targeted pre-training is essential for any child with profound global developmental delays. It is just as essential for the adult that dreads the idea of potty training. Once they begin targeted pre-training and see results, they replace dread with hope.

Henry was trying to pull down his sweatpants over a full and very stinky diaper. Danielle, his nanny, finished loading the dishwasher just in time to grab him before that diaper opened up. He wasn't the fastest at getting into the tub or climbing onto the bus, but he could be amazingly quick at undressing when he had a full diaper. What he lacked in coordination, he made up for in pure determination. Henry would keep at it until whatever he was wearing was off. If the diaper ripped and dumped out, he was oblivious to the mess it made. He was a free man, and off he would go!

She wished he was showing any interest in learning to use the potty. He wasn't. Danielle considered making him get a clean diaper from the shelf before she changed him. The first step would be stopping him from his plan to rip the full diaper off in the middle of the kitchen.

What are the benefits of pre-training?

Children who have been taught to be directly involved in their diapering, who have a vocabulary for elimination, and who can handle the natural frustration of learning a new sensory-motor skill have advantages when they start formal training. They are used to following simple directions and show patience when waiting for brief periods. Having already built some of the sensory processing and balance skills needed to sit on a toilet in a small space, they won't be as likely to fall down or fall apart. Pre-training makes it less common for a child to develop withholding behaviors due to fear of accidents or the desire for a power struggle. Kids that have experienced pre-training can more easily recover from toileting setbacks around extended school breaks or illness. Kids who have been pre-trained can handle changes in bathroom equipment or using new environments better.

Their caregivers receive benefits as well. They can anticipate some of the biggest potential problems for formal training before it begins. They also know what strengths a child has; these strengths will support them in learning and coping while they learn. In many cases, pre-training could reveal to caregivers that it is already time to start formal potty training. Adults who use pre-training know what the right equipment and the best clothes are for potty training this particular child. There won't be a frantic run to a store or a frantic search on a screen for these things. They know what categories of treats or non-edible rewards work best for the child. Caregivers have learned what the signs of waning motivation looks like and know how to turn it around. Because they have learned about their own strengths and limitations in pre-training, they can ask for support when things get tough. Parents and professionals that have done pre-training feel confident about what is ahead. Anyone who is uncertain that pre-training is important for success should think about how they felt before they had their first child or started their first job. They need to remember the conflicting information they found online, and how it felt to be stuck with a problem without a basket of tools. If they had acquired more practical information and had a chance to practice before jumping into their new role, their stress levels would have been lower and life would have been easier. They would still have been doing some very hard work. Preparation didn't eradicate the need for effort. Every adult wants a roadmap at the start of toilet training a hypotonic child. Pre-training is the way to draw some of the lines on that map.

In sales, there is an acronym: ABC. Whether selling tech services, a car, or a washing machine, it means "Always Be Closing (the sale)". Great salespeople are seamlessly weaving messaging about buying their product into their conversations and actions with customers. They make their customers feel like they are being helped, not being sold a product. If what they are selling is a product that their customer needs, the customer is indeed being helped. For pre-training, the "C" in "ABC" is changed to a "T". The adults using pre-training begin to think "Always Be Training" as they go through their day. They transform from being caretakers to being both teacher and caretaker. This isn't joylessly talking about pee or poop all the time. It isn't adding another task to an already busy day. It is mindfully using everyday actions to build the readiness skills a child with low muscle tone needs to get ready for formal potty training. Three ways to embody "ABT" are to use Potty Talk, Potty Models, and Potty Play. Let's take a look at each strategy, what they teach, and how to use them daily.

Potty Talk

The adults surrounding a child need to talk about the process and the products of elimination, which teaches them necessary vocabulary and to focus the child's attention on diaper changing. This can also be done by using sign language or graphic communication systems such as PECS (picture exchange communication system). Caregivers may not realize that a child who looks at a toy or a screen during a diaper change should instead be listening to <u>them</u> while they narrate the process. They might think that there is no point to describing what they are doing when there isn't any indication that it makes any difference to a child.

They would be wrong.

Tiffany wondered if James would ever be able to participate in diaper changes as easily as his little sister did. He had learned a few signs and was able to make eye contact with her when he wanted something he couldn't access by himself. He had made so much progress since starting to attend a therapeutic preschool program! When she changed his diaper, he didn't fight her unless he was very involved in watching a show. She had recently learned that if she allowed him to bring a car with him, he was calmer during diapering. But this meant he mostly ignored her. Did he show any awareness that he needed a diaper? Not as far as she could see. She tried to push the feelings of worry into the back of her mind. The day was young, and there were three full baskets of dirty clothes in front of her.

Potty talk during diapering doesn't makes the task take appreciably longer or require more physical effort. It can feel very one-sided at first, and it can feel that way unless you know how to look for signs that a child is beginning to understand, and even anticipate, what is said. The non-verbal indications of attention are when a child quiets their body slightly, turns toward the speaker, makes eye contact, uses reciprocal gaze, or vocalizes. It might be necessary to alter the style of "potty talk" with changes in tone or phrasing or add gestures to increase active listening. Making up a potty song adds rhythmicity and melody to the interaction. Anyone that has heard the national anthem or a religious song knows that music can shift attention and mood. If the style of potty talk is different from the adult's usual tone and phrasing, these actions trigger attention in children with very limited language ability. They know something special is happening. Reducing competition for attention from screens and other sources of sound and visual images makes it easier to use Potty Talk successfully. These devices should be turned off or placed on mute.

Interacting with a child by describing the actions and items used during diapering communicates the adult's interest and messages the importance of the task. Children that have an elimination vocabulary can devote more attention to the sensory, motor, and social components of toileting. They will be capable of using the right words to ask for help. They will respond faster to instructions or questions.
Adults who take the time in pre-training to experiment with vocal tone, phrasing, and phrase length, and word selections make a difference in a child's responses are making progress in developing the child's functional communication. The same is true for the use of pacing and exaggeration in the use of sign language, or the choice of images with PECS. Yes; the adult is the one who has changed during targeted pre-training. But there is no communication without first gaining the attention of your audience.

Parents will have to decide if they want to use anatomical and technical terms for body parts, functions, and elimination products or if they will use nicknames like "wee-wee" and "caca". It is more important to be consistent than to be scientifically correct. A child's team can work together to make the decision what vocabulary makes sense. Kids doing pre-training need to hear the same words for the same body parts and actions from every adult diapering and dressing them. Confusion about whether "do-do" and "poop" are the same thing will slow down learning. And of course, all "potty talk" should be appropriate for the child's age and developmental level.

Adults need to be honest with themselves about their comfort level for directly speaking about bodies and bodily functions. Remember; children with the most limited command of language will focus on the emotional content of our communication, not the words. Some parents feel strongly that using anatomically correct names for body parts creates children that aren't ashamed of their body, and children that can accurate report any abusive encounters are safer from predators. Other parents feel uncomfortable doing so and do not use anatomical names for body parts and actions with other adults or even medical providers. Some "potty talk" isn't about pee, poop, and diapers. It includes words for objects and prepositions. Improving a child's attention to directions for <u>any</u> self-care task will prepare them to learn toileting skills. It is not clear that vocabulary is the only or even the most powerful determinant of a child's bodily self-image and self-esteem. What is clear is that children need to be able to understand us and communicate effectively during toilet training to be successful. By practicing terms and building comfort levels in pre-training, adults and children can communicate with ease and clarity. When a child needs to run to the potty in formal training, they can state why and ask for the help they need.

One very important communication strategy that builds independent toileting is to shorten any verbal, signed, or PECS prompts as a child makes progress, eventually using very general cues or no language at all. This is contrary to standard speech therapy strategies to require and offer longer utterances in communication. A child who knows that they are expected to go to the shelf and get a clean diaper once they enter the changing area should not be told what to do any longer. If they forget or are distracted, reducing a prompt to a vague question like "Hmmm, uh-oh?" forces them to <u>think</u> about what has gone wrong or what they have forgotten. This is gradually preparing the child with low muscle tone to solve a problem in the bathroom independently.

Potty Models

Typical kids frequently wander into the bathroom while parents and siblings are using the toilet. They are often toileted in groups at daycare and pre-school, beginning around the ages of 2.5-3. They see and hear what other kids are told and what they are doing. Because typical children have so many opportunities for incidental learning, it is possible for the sibling of a pre-schooler to become toilet trained far more quickly than a hypotonic child. Few young children label bathroom use as "icky". Adults and older kids provide that label. They are far more curious than judgmental. A child that is unable to walk around the house or remains sitting more of their day may still be curious about toilet use. They may have never seen anyone use the toilet because by the time they arrive, the "deed" has been done.

Bella wandered into Sean and Luke's en-suite bathroom just as Sean was flushing the toilet. His underwear and pants were still down around his ankles. He was caught completely off-guard, because when he left the kitchen, she had been eagerly eating her way through a big breakfast. It had never occurred to him to close the bathroom door. "Oh, well" he thought, "It had to happen someday." Bella did not show any interest in her dad's half-naked body or the contents of the toilet. She grabbed his hand while staring at the top of his tall dresser in the bedroom. She was making it clear that what she wanted was his iPad, not an anatomy lesson. So much for any emerging curiosity about the "Why" or the "How" of using the toilet.

If a child with low muscle tone has shown no interest in bathroom activities, adults need to try taking the child into the bathroom next time "nature calls". They don't need to say much or force questions. Because of the intimacy of this situation, this pre-training activity is usually limited to the child's parents. When faced with a live demonstration, curiosity and questions can bloom. This personal invitation won't be extended to every bathroom visit. That doesn't mean that kids don't simmer with questions and ideas. They could have questions at the time they are in the bathroom, or later in the day or in a week. Those questions are signs of training readiness!

Targeted Potty Models includes demonstrating the skills related to using the toilet. Hand washing and drying, plus flushing a toilet (you can flush clean toilet paper!) are both essential skills. Frequent demonstrations of these skills, with or without narration, increases familiarity and provides details that typically developing kids take for granted. Some children are far more interested in watching their siblings use the toilet than watching their parents. Not all siblings feel comfortable with this, so parents need to be sensitive and not force anything.

Potty Play

Targeted pre-training doesn't have to be rigid or boring. Potty Play can make pre-training fun and creative. Play is a wonderful way to learn and practice toileting skills. Learning toileting vocabulary and the related motor skills can happen through play. In pre-training, the themes of play focus on what urgency feels like, clothing management, sitting on the toilet, and hygiene skills. Adults will have to be more directive in their play during Potty Play than they may be with other play philosophies. For example, if they are trained in the FloorTime model, this therapeutic strategy requires the adult to follow the child's lead. Potty Play and FloorTime can co-exist; they are done at different times of the child's day.

The adults provide toys and tools for play that are as close to the items a child will be using in formal toilet training. For example, they will use plastic dolls whose bottoms can be wiped with the same wipes the child will eventually use. Underwear that fits a child or can be put on a doll by a child might require a bigger doll or a large stuffed animal that has two legs and a waist. Using appealing tools raises interest, so it might be helpful to use a pair of superhero underwear, then pretend that the doll is using the toilet or needs a diaper change. Dolls that urinate water with a press of a button may be truly fascinating to children who have entered the imaginative play stage.

All play needs to be sensitive to a hypotonic child's needs and challenges to be successful. A child that has a serious sensory sensitivity may not enjoy cleaning up the water that comes out of a doll that wets. They might need assistance and reassurance. A sensory seeker may find cleaning and wiping up the mess to be so much fun that they want the doll to "wet" on everything! Some kids do not enjoy imaginative play. They find pretending that a stuffed animal needs to wear underwear frustrating, because it is not human, and only humans wear clothes. Always craft Potty Play to fit the child's needs. Some children, particularly rigid thinkers, resist using their dolls or stuffed animals in a new way. They could need some new toys for Potty Play. Children that need time to accept new things and new ideas should be given the chance to watch an adult play with a new toy without being encouraged IN ANY WAY to play with it. Cheerful demonstration without the demand to join in could be the single most helpful thing a parent or caregiver can do to encourage the use of a new toy. Not even making a casual offer. Nothing. Just an adult demonstrating a play schema and expressing how much fun they are having. Potty Play with a resistant child begins with frequent and brief opportunities, done at various times of the day. To develop a transitional play schema, a child's familiar play receives a brief addition of Potty Play and Potty Talk, and then their familiar play schema returns. This is the therapeutic "bookending" technique used to reduce anxiety around novelty. If a child has significant anxiety when Potty Play is started, the adult should clearly state when Potty Play is finished for the moment, the day, or the session.

Collaborative Diapering

In pre-training using Collaborative Diapering, a child still wears a diaper, and the adult still changes them when they get wet or soiled. The experience of the diaper change has been transformed. This is true for the child and the adult. Both the child and the adult will have new roles and actions <u>every time</u> a soiled or wet diaper gets changed.

Why?

Because this is pre-training. "Collaborative Diapering" means that the child's routine of passively looking at a screen or at the mobile above the changing table is over. This may start with simply paying attention to the adult as they narrate their actions. It will progress to assisting with every single step of diapering. This will build pre-training skills in even the most delayed child. Collaborative diapering is a more focused teaching experience embedded in everyday caretaking. A child is asked to participate and assisted to do so. Their participation is recognized using focused attention, praise, or tangible rewards. As a child becomes more involved, the adult will add a new task for the child to do during diapering to increase their level of independence.

Even if no other component of pre-training has been used by the time formal training is attempted, collaborative diapering alone will develop many of the readiness skills for potty training. Without collaborative diapering and pre-training, doing formal toilet training with a hypotonic child is an uphill journey on a good day.

Tiffany had been working on her pre-training ideas for both Olivia and Andy. Her focus lately had been on getting them to participate in diapering plus learning the vocabulary. Olivia was her test subject, because her reactions to Tiffany were more visible and consistent. She scooped up Olivia and snuggled her for a moment. "Hiya, sweetie! Time for a fresh diapee!" Olivia was absolutely oblivious to the smell coming from her very full diaper.

Tiffany was not. She couldn't wait for both of her kids to be trained. The smell of poop made her more nauseous with every single diaper change. She had always been sensitive to foul smells. Her deep love for both of her kids had not changed that reaction one tiny bit! It had been the hardest thing to get used to after giving birth to James. She had researched early potty training when he was younger. James had been diagnosed with ASD shortly after her initial online research. Her hopes of early training had evaporated at that moment. But she was starting to think this "collaborative diapering" thing was do-able.

Olivia just smiled as she was lifted onto the changing table, and she pulled on Tiffany's hair with a few chubby fingers. With practiced precision, her mom slipped down Olivia's leggings. She chanted "Pants go down, down, DOWN." Tiffany handed Olivia a new diaper while she got out the wipes and diaper rash cream. She thought that Olivia could end up chewing the wipes or squish out the cream, but she wanted her to be playing with something to do with diaper changes. Tiffany gave her the wipes and she promptly dropped them on her belly. The tube of diaper cream was more interesting to her. Olivia looked briefly at the picture of the smiling baby on the tube, then switched to looking at her mom.
Tiffany smiled and said directly into her daughter's sweet little face "OK, hon, tooshie UP!", and Olivia popped her behind up like a little drawbridge. She giggled in response to the silly voice her mother used to say the word "UP". Tiffany removed the wet diaper, wiped her, and slid a fresh diaper under Olivia. Then

she told Olivia "Tooshie DOWN", and Olivia quickly dropped her behind onto the clean diaper so it could be fastened securely.

They went through the "UP and DOWN" routine again as Tiffany got her leggings back up. When she was done, she told Olivia "Time for trash" and placed her daughter on the floor. She handed her the wrapped diaper, and the toddler walked over to the Diaper Genie. Olivia opened the top and placed it inside. This was her second favorite part of the diapering routine. The high-5 before they left her room was what she loved the most.

Tiffany realized that she had not required Olivia to come into the bedroom where the changing table was located. She had carried her there. Her plan for the next diaper change would be to ask Olivia to walk with her to the bedroom and stand next to the table. Maybe Olivia could start helping her slide her pants down. That might be easier with something other than Lycra leggings…

Collaborative diapering is a learning experience for parents, caregivers, and professionals. They are paying attention to when and how often soiled or wet diapers occur in a typical day. This teaches them about a child's physiologic readiness for potty training, and how different types of meals or activities alter digestion and kidney function. They will have a better idea of when to take a child to the toilet later in training. They see which gestures and words improve cooperation, and which ones create frustration and defiance.

It will become easier to know if a lack of cooperation is because a child is exhausted or if they are tuning an adult out. If being hugged for tossing the soiled diaper out puts a smile on a child's face, they know that physical affection could be a strong reward in formal training. If failing to get the diaper in the trash 3 times brings on a tantrum, an adult knows initial successes need to be easier to achieve.

By altering the diapering routine to resemble the interactions, the environment, and the physical activities associated with using the toilet, formal training will not feel so foreign to either party. This is where pre-training becomes magical. A child who is lying down for a diaper change can learn to lift their hips on request when the adult is removing or putting a diaper on them. Some kids will try to wipe their genitals. Unless this creates an unreasonable mess, they should be allowed to do so. This doesn't mean that they are capable of effectively cleaning their body. They are beginning to learn the sequence of actions and the motor control for future independence.

Jordan had explained to her nanny Danielle that she wanted her son to be more involved in the process. Danielle decided to focus on getting to Henry before Henry could get to his full diaper. Every time. This meant that she had to pay a lot more attention to him. Responding to her group texts would have to wait until he was napping. And so would her cousin, who wanted her to call and talk her through a messy divorce. Danielle now had a messy <u>diaper</u> to deal with, and her cousin would simply have to wait until later to tell her about the recent dust-up with her ex. Luckily, the odor coming from Henry's backside helped alert her almost immediately to the situation. She left the laundry in the washer and ignored her phone. Whoever it was would have to wait.

Danielle guided Henry to the bathroom. He was clearly still in "removal" mode, so she took advantage of it. She had been told to get him involved in the process. So she did. Danielle pulled the front of the waistband away from his belly and placed his right hand on top. He immediately pushed the waistband down. She pulled the back of the pants down, and they dropped to his ankles. Danielle was a lot more involved in getting him on the changing table and taking off the full diaper. Henry's hands would be inside it if she did not act quickly. So she did. But she wrapped it up carefully by the adhesive tabs, so Henry could carry it to the trash when he was changed and she put him on the floor.

If a child doesn't complete any pre-training actions, the adult should not immediately speak or take any action. This allows time for noticing that the action has stopped. When nothing at all is happening, it might cause them to realize that they are the reason! A non-responsive child may need repeated instruction or assistance to complete their part of diapering. The adult will take over the child's job only when the child's actions risk their safety or when they become too agitated to participate. The child is wearing a diaper, there is no rush to manage clothing quickly. This helps a child to be more active during diaper changes and eventually more independent during formal toilet training.

Collaborative Diapering 2.0: pit-stop precision and more confidence for all

Refining pre-training skills includes making a child more independent, faster, and able to perform a series of actions. It may not happen naturally. Kids with low muscle tone are still kids who have spent their lives dependent on adults for so much. Parents and caregivers often need to set things up for advanced Collaborative Diapering to develop. Giving fewer prompts, asking for completion of multi-step instructions rather than performing a single step, and asking for more initiation. These are only a few of the easy ways to refine a child's pre-training skills. A child that needs to be told to toss their soiled-but-wrapped diaper in the trash is now handed the diaper without a prompt. The child that awkwardly pulls their pants down on one side of their hips now uses both hands at the same time and slide their pants down below their knees independently. When a child can walk into the bathroom and has formed bowel movements, it is time for both the adult and the child to go into the bathroom and carefully dump the contents of their diaper into the toilet while the child watches. Children can be told that "This is where the poop goes when big kids and grownups use the toilet" and allow them to help with flushing.

Pre-training skills that were only used at home can now be taken on the road! Doing collaborative diapering only at home teaches a child that participation in diapering is optional. That is a concept that breed resistance, withholding, and defiance. Parts of collaborative diapering can be used outside the changing room or bathroom. A child in advanced Collaborative Diapering is expected to completely wash and dry their hands at home, school, and at their relative's homes. Refining pre-training is essential to perform if there are any breaks or pauses in formal toilet training. When formal training resumes, the child who has refined their pre-training skills will show faster progress than they did at the beginning of training!

Chapter 5

Building Balance and Stability for Toileting

Jordan caught Henry as he slowly slid off the toilet and she blocked his exit from the bathroom. She needed to wipe his bottom before he ran out naked and stinky, eager to grab her suddenly unsupervised iPhone off the kitchen island. He almost always wobbled when he was sitting on the toilet, but he never worried about how close his face got to the edge of the vanity top. And once he was off the toilet, he felt free to leave, clean or not.

Jordan would never forget the time his face connected with the sharp corner of that vanity's edge. "Oh, don't worry. Head and face wounds always bleed way more than you'd think!" the PA cheerfully told her that night at pediatric urgent care. She was grateful that the PA was so calm as he sewed up Henry's cheek that night. She certainly had <u>not</u> been calm. All the blood, and the screams, and the chaos of that night, would never fully leave her memory.

Her ex, Lewis, had to be texted and informed of the injury. He routinely took the opportunity to remind her of that night whenever they fought. She was certain she had only looked at her watch for a second. It was in that second Henry decided to slide off of the toilet.

Toilet transfers

Occupational and physical therapists teach children to sequence the movements involved in approaching the potty, turning to stand or sit, carefully sitting down if needed, and then all the moves needed to get back up and turn around again. They refer to such movements as "transfers". To get safely on and off the toilet, a child needs strength and endurance, but also enough balance and stability so they don't fall while turning and bending. They need to pay attention to their environment and how they are moving. Anyone who has tripped when their phone rings knows that this is true. Children

77

with low muscle tone vary widely in their strength, coordination, endurance, and balance skills. The rubber meets the road when they need to gather these skills together with thinking and emotions and perform in the bathroom. Every time parents and therapists work on a PT or OT home exercise program, they are helping their child develop the ability to be safer, faster, and to move with better control. Exploring exactly how their exercises align with building the skills needed for toilet training is faster when parents…ask the therapists! A child's therapists can answer these questions and they can give an update on progress. When parents know why these exercises matter it can be motivation to persist with them. Parents and caregivers can think of it like training the child for a marathon: the marathon of toilet training.

James liked to hold Jacqueline's hand while he sat on the potty. She thought it was sweet, and a sign that he loved her. This meant a lot to Jacqueline, who felt a strong heart connection with her grandson. What Jacqueline did not realize was that James was using Jacqueline's hand as a grab bar that would also act as a safety net. He sensed, correctly, that she would catch him if he wobbled. He also used her as a distraction from the echo in the bathroom, and as entertainment. He watched her and smiled more when she sang a song. When she saw him smile she would keep singing "Itsy Bitsy Spider"; his favorite!

Children with low tone can get into a habit of searching for physical support in any location they can find it. They could lean on a person or lean on a piece of furniture for support. This continues while they sit on the potty. They also expect to be caught before they fall. Both need to change to achieve independent toileting. During toilet training, children must be personally responsible for balancing while they eliminate and manage clothing, wiping, and flushing. There is a distinction between having balance and using current skills to maintain safety with toileting: a child may not need to improve their balance skills to improve their performance! Some kids do not optimize their current skills in functional situations. Leaning on objects or people outside of toileting may not have any consequences, practical or social. Requesting help may be far easier than taking time and attention for safety and sequencing movements. The environment they are in could be too complex or too difficult for them to use their balance skills. But with using the toilet independently, it is time for a child to know which surfaces are safe choices, and when adapting movements are a better choice than seeking a support surface. This is best learned through practice in real life environments. In bathrooms.

Adults will need good observational skills to identify whether a child is able to balance well in one location but not another, with one adult but not others, or with one motivator (peer pressure, praise, or rewards, etc.) and not others. For children with low muscle tone, something as simple as wearing their orthotics and shoes can be all the difference between needing to lean and being able to stand and transfer safely.
The adult's job is to gradually move from direct assistance and adapting the environment to using verbal and physical cues, then finally allowing a child to be fully responsible for their safety during toileting. Because providing physical support may be unconsciously linked into beliefs about what a "good" parent or caretaker does, both the child and the adult have to adjust their mindset as well as their actions. Explaining to a child that they now must use the safest way to move, not the fastest, could be a true shift in thinking. Their therapists have always emphasized safe independent movement, but that may not be true at school or at home. Adults want a child to be safe. They don't always communicate to a child that they also have responsibility for their own safety. And adults don't always administer consequences when those responsibilities are ignored. Holding a child accountable in some way, and turning a bad choice into a teachable moment, takes planning and practice. This can be as simple as asking a child to repeat their transfer with greater safety. This means that they can't run out of the bathroom to finish watching a show or get back in the pool. It is a small consequence, but it can be meaningful. It messages how important moving safely is. If safe transfers seems to be harder than they should be, any teacher or parent can request help from the child's physical or occupational therapist treating a hypotonic child can help. It can even become an IEP goal.

Using the toilet is complicated by one unique balance issue that doesn't crop up with other types of transfers: clothing is only partially removed during toileting. Pants, skirts, and underwear have to be managed safely. Figuring out when and how to manage clothing before, during, and after using the toilet is an essential skill. It also makes moving harder. Children need to be positioned to sit (or stand) before they move clothing. They must replace clothing before they step away from the toilet and wash their hands. In between, clothes can't get in the way of urinating or defecating or there will be a mess to clean up.

Well-meaning caregivers might conclude that toileting naked will increase safety. Some kids think this too! Unfortunately, it is not a good idea to strip a child's clothes off completely before getting them on the toilet. It delays access to the potty long enough to risk an accident, setting a child up for failure. Clothes must also be put back on in every situation unless the child is in the middle of a "boot camp" week.

Completing the correct sequence of movements during a transfer is crucially important. Lowering pants before turning or dropping a skirt down before wiping won't work. Children with low muscle tone often choose less-than-optimal movement sequences. They try to skip steps or combine them to move more quickly or preserve their balance. Kids need to be in a position that will allow them to either remain standing to urinate or to sit on the toilet <u>after</u> they have positioned their clothes. They must be balanced enough to reach to their thighs or knees to wipe, then retrieve underwear or pants without falling over. Reaching behind their body to control clothing or wipe while maintaining their balance can be harder than reaching forward.

Some children have footprint outlines drawn on their footstool. They place their feet inside the outline once the footstool is centered in front of the toilet or the sink. If needed, a PECS system can be mounted next to the toilet as a guide. Some families decide installing a grab bar is easier than prompting or making the trip to Urgent Care. A grab bar installed next to the toilet serves as both a physical assist as well as a visual and spatial cue. Children use the bar to steady their body with one hand while pulling clothes up or down with their other hand. They don't need to hold it for it to work: the position of the grab bar is a cue "tells" them where to sit or stand. Use of an adaptive device instead of an adult can stimulate greater independence in a child that tends to rely on assistance whenever it is available.

A quick comment about positioning for boys: kids that stand while urinating have to do three things at once. They need to balance while releasing the external urinary sphincter and while directing the stream of urine into the toilet bowl or the urinal. In the beginning, it can be harder for them to do all three things at the same time. Some boys need a <u>lot</u> of practice and reminders. Some need to use a grab bar to accomplish this. Many parents want to begin potty training by teaching their sons to urinate in sitting. They believe that it is less confusing for a child to sit for both urination and bowel movements. They could be right. The problems begin when they do not know how to transition their child into standing to urinate. Anatomically, standing to urinate is easier for almost every boy. Once they are standing to urinate, visual attention can wander. This could be a poor choice, because their urine stream will follow their body's direction, which often follows the path of their gaze! If a child with very limited control insists on standing, then they need more supervision plus a good reason to focus on the task "at hand". Aiming their urine stream at cereal bits floating in the toilet bowl could be that reason. As a bonus, kids want to hydrate more, the better to have "ammo" to play this game! Helping to clean up accidents could be that reason. Deducting the amount of time it takes to clean from a timed treat such as screen use could also be very motivating.

When sitting is the problem

Some parents, teachers, and caregivers find that they don't have much of a chance to figure out if a child is unsteady or unsure of how to sit down on the toilet; the child isn't willing to sit long enough to assess their sitting balance! Kids that balk at sitting on the toilet or potty seat always have a reason. There isn't another seat in the house (or the school) that has a hole in the center. This makes the toilet seat look and feel unfamiliar. Assisting with dumping the poop from their diaper into the toilet in Collaborative Diapering should have demonstrated what toilets are for. Washing their hands in the bathroom and practicing flushing a piece of toilet paper or a few colored cereal circles (they get to pick their color and eat a few if they wish!) are two additional ways to become more familiar with toilets. Dry Runs also give kids brief practice at sitting on a toilet seat and getting familiar with how it feels.
Unless the seat is too wobbly, too small, or too large for a child, they are un-

likely to think they will fall in. There are two exceptions. A child that has visual deficits, or severe visual-perceptual limitations, could be truly afraid. The ability to judge depth requires coordination of both eyes together. Low muscle tone can affect eye muscles too. A child with poor depth perception either sees double or shuts down information from one eye when they look at something. These kids always have some degree of motor challenge during toddlerhood. They avoid early ball play and move more cautiously through the world. They may even close their eyes when it would seem logical to open them. Fortunately, there are vision therapies that can improve depth perception, and adaptive strategies to support a child feeling safe while using the toilet.

Bella had always had a "lazy eye". The ophthalmologist wasn't certain she would put up with patching and was against using eye drops, so they tried surgery. It did work, at first. Then that eye started to drift in the other direction. She was scheduled for another surgery in a few months. Sean and Luke crossed their collective fingers that the second one would fix this. In the meantime, they wondered if her fear of stepping off the curb and her slow descent on the stairs were connected to her eye problems.

The other exception that creates realistic fear of sitting on the toilet is the child who struggles with the sensation of changing their head out of a vertical position. They may have learned to climb onto an adaptive chair at school or at home, or half-fall or crash onto furniture in their home. It may be physically possible to sit on a toilet, but the movements make them feel dizzy or disoriented. Getting on and off a toilet (which is a seat without arms to hold or padding to cushion their landing) is much harder for them. These kids will need more practice and may need grab bars installed in the bathroom they will use for training. Many schools have a similar training bathroom. Asking the staff at their school if they can practice toilet transfers is a reasonable request to improve a child's confidence.

If the seat is stable and fits them well, it is much more likely that most kids that resist sitting on the toilet have other things that are stressing them out. It may not be immediately evident, but they do have a reason. Possibly more than one.

Kids who have terrific balance and can sit on a fence rail with ease aren't likely to be afraid to fall into the toilet if the seat fits them well. They may be confused about why they are sitting on a new seat, or why they are sitting in a room without any toys or a screen to watch. Children who don't like the way the seat feels on bare skin or how the sounds echo off tiled walls aren't afraid of the toilet. They are stressed by the sensory experiences of sitting half-naked. If a child has no idea why they were asked to stop playing and has been placed in a small room, they may be protesting from confusion and frustration, not from fear.

Because children's pants are pulled down to their ankles when they are helped onto the toilet, and an adult is encouraging them to remain sitting, it is obvious to a child that cooperation with sitting means staying put until told to leave. A child that is used to moving around freely without limitations will find this stressful. They may be able to sit at school, but not at home. Using a visual timer or hourglass may not make a difference if this is the first situation in which they have been asked to sit passively outside of school without being in a car seat.

Pre-training emphasizes activities that build a child's ability to follow directions and gain some patience. Readers who want to know how to grow a child's patience for sitting as well as building patience for everything else in life can flip to chapter 9 and read about Dr. Harvey Karp's truly amazing Patience Stretching technique.

Dry Runs

One of the most successful methods to build independence, speed, and safety in toilet transfers (as well as clothing management) before formal toilet training is to do Dry Runs. This pun is very much intended! The child practices approaching the toilet, turning, and sitting or standing to pee, standing back up from sitting, then turning to "pretend flush", all while fully dressed. Transfer-focused Dry Runs break the experience down (no pants around their ankles, no wiping) to make it easier to learn. There is no urgency to sit quickly for elimination. When a child has mastered transfers, they can combine transfer Dry Runs and wiping/dressing Dry Runs. Dry Runs can be turned into a game with incentives or incorporated into Potty Play. A child gets a sticker for their chart for repeating the Dry Run sequence 10 times, or their doll takes turns with the child. The doll can make all the mistakes, or it can model the correct actions, the most fun option wins.

A hypotonic child also needs balance and stability to stand in front of the toilet or the sink to perform flushing, washing, and drying their hands. Reaching the lever to flush requires some balance. So does reaching the towel on the bar or hook. An adult will probably be assisting with these actions initially to ensure good hygiene. They are watching out for safety as well. If the soap and the towels need to be moved to a better location prior to formal toilet training, learning this during Dry Runs is the best time to find it out. Standing safely on a footstool's small surface while using soap and water is a skill that requires practice. Adequate balance and safety as a child gets into position on a footstool is the most important component of this transfer. The Baby Bjorn footstool is the most stable and widely available footstool. A wobbly or slippery footstool is a mistake that can have serious consequences. Many kids like to wash their hands because they love to play with the suds and splash around in the sink. This can get out of hand and end up with the floor or footstool too wet to be safe. Setting a timer has helped many a child limit water play, as has a fun reason to leave the bathroom like playing outside.

Chapter 6

Selecting The Right Equipment for Toilet Training

Parents don't always know if they have the right equipment for potty training their hypotonic child. They might assume that a standard toilet, the toilet seat insert their older child used, or a toddler potty seat will work, without trying them out. In some instances, their poorly fitting toilet training equipment is a bigger problem than the child's low muscle tone. It is easy to miss the signs that the equipment is the problem. A child's agitation, refusal, or their frequent accidents could be blamed on their diagnosis by professionals as well as caregivers. Being new to doing toilet training doesn't help. A relatively inexperienced "potty coach", parent or professional, is more likely to assume that negative behavior has its origin in emotion or from a medical reason. The true cause could also be a bad fit between the child and their potty tools.

Getting it right once doesn't mean that equipment selection decisions are over. Defining what the best equipment is for a particular child will change as they make progress through potty training. The more physically challenged a child is, the more likely that their equipment needs change over time. Being prepared to upgrade or remove equipment as needed is as important as knowing how to get the right items to start toilet training. This chapter explains how to pick the right equipment for the job, and how to use equipment easily and successfully.

The goals of equipment selection are relatively simple: a child needs to be comfortable, stable, use the equipment as independently as possible for their stage of training, and be safe throughout the process. Equipment selection begins with which toilet to use. Should a child use an adult toilet with modifications; all children eventually need to make the switch to the adult toilet? Should they start with potty seats, and if so, which one and where should potty seats be located? Do they need more than one in a home?

85

Using a standard toilet depends on the child's size and if they can sit with enough comfort and stability independently or if they need a seat insert or a footstool. An insert creates a smaller opening for a child to achieve stable sitting. A footstool gives a child the ability to climb onto the toilet seat then place their feet firmly. Footstools are not only for reaching the potty or the sink. Kids who can place their feet firmly on a surface, allowing their knees to be slightly above the height of their hips, can activate their core to increase intra-abdominal pressure during bowel movements: they can help push the poop out.

Equipment choice also depends on what is realistic for the home/school environment. Some home bathrooms have no available floor space to add a potty seat. Some preschools install child-sized toilets. A family may consider this choice for a bathroom in their home that the child will frequently use. One advantage to using a standard toilet, with or without other items, is that this eliminates the need to change equipment later in the process of training. Removing a seat insert can be less disruptive or confusing for them than switching the strategies to get on and off different equipment.

Smaller children need a seat insert for safety while sitting on a standard toilet. Stable seat inserts that have been permanently attached to a toilet don't slide while sitting or when moving from standing to sitting. This stability gives children a sense of safety and focus attention on other issues. Seat inserts with handles have the same effect for kids who need them. Many children with low tone, and particularly those that have sensory sensitivities, are more comfortable using a padded seat insert. These retain a small amount of body heat, making a child's bare skin more comfortable. Padded seats also reduce the chance that skin will not stick or become slippery from sweat after prolonged sitting. Both sticking to the seat or slipping while sitting on the toilet can increase fall risk.

Lewis stared at the choices for toilet seat inserts online. Potty inserts with handles, without handles, padded, unpadded, and folding. His eyes started crossing. He had no idea if any of them would fit on the upstairs toilet, and if he needed one for the powder room toilet too. Maybe he could use a potty seat in the main floor powder room instead? Henry was 4 but small for his age. He searched the online comments for clues and advice.

Asking his ex-wife Jordan was a non-starter. She always took every available opportunity to tell him that he didn't know as much as she did about or about Henry. In the 3 years they had been divorced, her sharp comments on his opinions about both subjects had been quite consistent. Lewis knew that they should be on the same page. Every article he read on special needs parenting when you are divorced said so. He understood it. He just didn't know how to accomplish it.

His mother Sharon would love to take over the job of picking out bathroom equipment. "She would love to take over <u>everything</u> about Henry's life" thought Lewis. He knew that asking Sharon for advice would make his life easier in the moment, and his life as a co-parent a lot harder. Jordan would reject anything Sharon picked out, just because it was Sharon's choice. Back to the online comments section...

Should a child use a potty seat rather than a toilet?

Potty seats can be great choices for younger or smaller children. A potty seat sits directly on the floor, allowing a child to place their feet firmly on the floor. Accidentally falling off or tipping over a potty seat is practically impossible. Children who are extremely fearful of falling off a standard toilet or who are unsafe using a footstool may need to use a potty seat while they develop the skills and confidence needed to use a standard toilet and footstool. Some potty seats have arm rests or handles. They are portable and affordable, easy to clean. There are a wide range of potty seat choices and features.
Placing a potty seat on every floor of a large home can reduce accidents if a child needs extra time to make it to the potty. There is a risk. Placing potty seats in living spaces instead of bathrooms weakens the message that elimination should happen in bathrooms. Making the decision about where to place potty seats should be made on a case-by-case basis, while working hard on skills like clothing management, diet, communication, and building willingness to follow adult cues.

Sean decided to buy two items; a removable seat insert with padding and handles that said it fit all styles of toilet seats, and a screw-on toilet seat that was two toilet seats in one. Bella wouldn't be able to fling that one! That seat wasn't padded though, and it had no handles. It would go in the downstairs half bath that Maggie would be using with her during the day. Maggie had no patience for Bella's throwing behaviors. She was a great caregiver, and he and Luke had decided that they would try hard not to make potty training a reason for her to give up.

If there is no floor space to place a potty seat in a bathroom, it may not be a realistic option. Having a bathroom so small that the potty seat becomes a tripping hazard is not safe. Some families bounce between equipment in desperation as they encounter defiance or the child's progress slows. Thoughtful planning and an understanding of toilet training will prevent this frantic behavior. Children, even children with cognitive limitations, can perceive that their parents are upset, and that using the toilet is the problem.

The biggest problem with potty seats when compared to toilet inserts? Older kids or larger toddlers don't fit well on these seats. They are always designed for toddlers. Even if older children are slim, they are sitting with their knees much higher than their hips. This is an awkward position, and using the potty seat can be rejected outright for that reason alone. It is also difficult to sit down and stand up from a very low position, increasing the amount of time a child needs to begin to use a potty seat. An older child can tip over a low potty seat as they try to get up and down, creating a mess and provoking agitation in the child as well as the caregiver who cleans up the mess! Older boys who are urinating in sitting may not have enough room to direct their stream. These accidents could have been expected and avoided by fitting the toilet to the child.

Some potty seats are slightly adjustable in height by altering the height of the base. It needs to be wide and strong enough to bear the weight of a child easily. Caregivers should never place a potty seat on a small footstool or on a box. This is unstable. Even with supervision, using an unstable set-up places a child in a risky position. When a child becomes frightened with seat movement during use, they could refuse to continue all training. Perception is reality. Parents or caregivers who aren't sure if an older child is too tall for a potty seat can ask a child's therapists to observe sitting and standing actions in person or from a video.

Finally, children look to adults to tell them if a situation is safe or not. Parents and caregivers that demonstrate confidence and show children how important their safety is in toilet training are messaging a value as well as a standard. The adults doing toilet training need to feel certain that the equipment being used is safe and say so. Out loud. Repeatedly. And provide details about why it is safe.

Cathy Collyer, OTR, LMT

Chapter 7

Building Sensory Processing for Toilet Training

Children with low muscle tone frequently have sensory processing difficulties that make potty training more challenging. Sensory processing issues were described in some detail in chapter One. It is ideal to address sensory processing issues in a practical manner during targeted pre-training. But life is complicated, and it may be necessary to work on sensory processing issues during formal training too. Using the toilet is a complex sensory-motor task. That is a fact. It does not mean that waiting for a child to have better sensory processing is the right choice. While sensory processing treatment is likely to make toilet training easier, it is possible to successfully navigate pre-training and even build functional sensory processing skills without intensive sensory treatment. Increasing opportunities to use a child's existing sensory skills and making the toileting environment and materials more sensory-friendly doesn't replace therapy; it supports the child's abilities at a particular time and place.

This is an important message for readers who are not occupational therapists (they know this stuff already!): a child's sensory processing can improve <u>in the moment</u> when the adults around them alter their actions and interactions to support better processing, and when their environment supports them to optimize their sensory processing <u>in that moment</u>.

Pre-training is the time for parents, teachers, and caregivers to learn how to touch and speak with a child for improved sensory processing, and how their gestures and other body movements affect a child's neurological activation. It is also the time to make sensory-aware bathroom adaptations so they can become familiar and be accepted before being needed in formal training. Parents and caregivers who have a better appreciation of a child's sensory pro-

91

cessing issues have developed a useful skill set. They can separate out a child's behavioral, cognitive, and communication challenges from sensory-based reactions. This means they will be able to respond more effectively when difficulties arise. An adult who can sense and respond effectively will also display greater compassion to the child. They remain confident during those periods of struggle and surf through plateaus in progress.

Knowing when to use the toilet is due to efficient sensory awareness and discrimination. We correctly interpret what is happening in our bodies as elimination urgency. We know these sensations are not an indication of danger, and they do not overwhelm us. But that is not the only type of sensory processing we do as we use the toilet. It includes smelling the products of elimination, the soaps in the room, touching our body to move clothing, wash, and wipe. It is balancing safely and focusing our vision to locate the materials we need to wipe and wash. During all of these sensory experiences, we remain alert and focused, but not overwhelmed.

Sensory Processing Challenges during Toileting

The child with sensory sensitivity isn't simply more aware of the smells, sounds, and textures in their body and in the bathroom. They have neurologically defensive responses. Their nervous system is messaging that they are under threat. Kids that are sensory seekers can find lots of sensory stimulation in a bathroom. Often so much that they forget what they are there to do! Lots of things to touch and explore…and distract them or dysregulate them! Children with poor sensory modulation may be unable to "wake up" enough or unable to calm down. The easily overwhelmed child struggles to calm down rapidly after being activated by the experience of using the bathroom. The under-responder can also struggle to get sufficiently activated enough to attend to signals for elimination urgency and respond quickly.

One way to manage many types of sensory processing challenges is to train a child to use the bathroom efficiently. This reduces the amount of sensory stimulation the sensory sensitive, sensory seeking, and overwhelmed modulator has to manage. Building skills like hand washing and clothing management in as well as outside of the bathroom makes a significant difference in how quickly a hypotonic child can use the bathroom. Efficiency reduces their frustration and confusion. Both frustration and confusion reduce sensory processing. Children use the bathroom more frequently during potty training. This is magnified when using the "boot camp" intensive process. Any pre-training that increases a child's ability to spend less time in the bathroom and decreases the stress of sensory processing will be very helpful for a child with sensory processing issues.

Henry never did well in elevators or narrow hallways. His OT thought it had a lot to do with his sound sensitivity. Corey, his dad, thought it had more to do with having fewer escape routes! Both of Corey's bathrooms in his condo were small. The powder room downstairs could only be described as "tiny". After child support payments, he had very little left at the middle of the month, let alone at the end of the month. Moving to a more spacious home was off the table for now. If Henry couldn't handle being changed in the bathroom downstairs during pre-training, Corey would have to bring him upstairs to the full bath. The chance of Henry "holding it" that long was slim. Corey felt tired just thinking about all of it. But if he bailed on this and didn't participate in pre-training, his ex would have a great excuse to ask him about his commitment to the plan and to his son. His own guilt would take care of any painful emotional points that his ex, Jordan, missed.

No other room in the home is as sensory-intense as the bathroom. Not even the kitchen. And not in a good way, for most kids. Filled with tile, running water, vent fans and more, most bathrooms have minimal soundproofing and maximal sound production in a small space. The smells, sounds, and the confined spatial experience of a bathroom can be overwhelming for sensory sensitive kids and sensory seekers alike. Poor sensory modulators who are easily overwhelmed might look fine going into the bathroom, and not so terrific leaving the bathroom.

Bella was a card-carrying sensory seeker. She had always been this way; her parents noticed it when she was a baby. Luke was not a sensory seeker, and he found her joy in exploring all types of sensations hard to understand. Bella had

93

no problems with the smells and sounds in the bathroom as he changed her diaper. Paying attention to anything he said or did was another thing. If she spotted the foam soap or could grab a fluffy towel first, she would rub her face with the towel and try to pump out as much of the soap as possible with glee, regardless of what else was happening. She could be in the middle of pulling up her pants with his help. That would be abandoned to play with anything she could find. Sima, Bella's OT, had suggested the foam soap because it would be easier to hold than a bar of soap. "Clearly", Luke thought, "Sima hasn't realized how well Bella's fine motor skills have progressed!"

Hypotonic kids who are sensory seekers can have poor sensory awareness of the sensations of urgency and what happens during toileting. Building interoceptive awareness for toilet training is a combination of educating a child on what subtle sensations exist and helping them understand how to respond to them correctly and promptly. Creating habits that minimize mistakes in registration and discrimination are useful. This could mean that after breakfast, their attention cannot be gripped too tightly on a screen or on a book. They will miss the signal to go pee or poop. Kids need practice to tune into their body's cues. They need to learn words that make sense to them, such as "full" or pressure", and use them correctly. Many kids with low tone need to stand up to take advantage of gravity's effect on a full bladder (greater pressure) and release their body weight from the pudendal nerve in their groin. A full bladder and colon is easier to feel when standing, and particularly so when moving around. Habits like using the bathroom before leaving the house or starting to play outside regardless of urgency cues are good choices. This will reduce their need to run to the bathroom in the middle of something fun. Physical therapy to build more core strength is helpful for some kids, but a strong core without a comprehensive toileting plan does not always result in fewer accidents.

Adapting the bathroom experience for sensory success

Reducing any unnecessary distractions in the bathroom helps everyone. It supports sensory-sensitive kids, sensory seekers, and children with poor sensory modulation. Sensitive kids, or children who are poor modulators and have hit their "wall", will be calmer and more focused. Sensory seekers won't have to work to suppress their desire to explore. They can focus better. Poor sensory modulators who can't come back down to baseline won't have to work so hard to get there.

Identifying when environments are affecting a particular child requires some skill. It can be as challenging for the adults to do this as it is for the child they are toilet training. Even highly skilled occupational therapists can fail to anticipate the delayed impact of a large cheerfully colored painting over the toilet on a poor sensory modulator. Some of that is inexperience, and some is the brief nature of therapy sessions. If the child's therapist doesn't see the precursors to a meltdown, they haven't seen the "whole show". Unless they ask more questions, they might never connect the dots. Parents and teachers may have to provide more details for teachers and therapists that haven't inquired enough to hear the whole story.

Not every bathroom sensory trigger is obvious. Conversations in the bathroom can be a source or sensory stimulation. These discussions could be about toileting. They could also be about other things, because kids may be sitting on the toilet for a while waiting to complete a bowel movement. If no one is thinking about focusing, the embroidered dolphin on a hand towel could produce a long and distracting discussion about dolphin communication, rather than allow a child to attend to urgency signals. Adults can lower their vocal volume, use fewer and shorter sentences, producing greater empty and calming airtime. Changing vocal tone and phrasing are effective ways to alter another person's neurological activation. Softer tones are calming. Sharper tones alert a child who is under-responsive. Children who are non-verbal or minimally verbal may have a better and faster response to alterations in volume, phrasing, and tone than verbal kids. They are used to tuning into these non-language cues to understand what is being said.

Decreasing the sensory stimulation caused by the physical environment can be accomplished by removing unneeded items and turning excessive fans and lights off or down. Musical timers are fun for some kids, but not every child can handle them. Turning their volume down or having firm rules about when they are used might help. Stashing non-essential items in cabinets or in portable baskets makes for a simpler visual scene and a neater space. Kids that need to increase their alertness need brighter lights and cooler air. The sound distortions in a bathroom can lead to a subtle level of irritation and distractibility, even anger. The same could happen with a child that has sensory sensitivity or sensory modulation issues that lead them to be unable to relax after being activated. White noise could mask some of the more irritating sounds. Adding sound-absorbing panels are another adaptation. The Sound Silencer panels from acousticsurfaces.com are an effective choice.

An adult can also limit their gestures and movements to those that highlight the task the child is performing in the moment. It can be very difficult to inhibit the desire to "multitask" and neaten up the bathroom or check texts. When it is clear how distracting it can be to a child with sensory processing challenges, it gets easier. It might seem like a "free" moment to quickly send a response before needing to supervise transfers and wiping. It isn't.

Luke thought that even though Bella wasn't his biological child, they had a lot more in common than Sean and Bella did, particularly around sensory processing. He did hate the sound of the toilet flushing, and the way voices echoed in a bathroom. He became anxious; she got disorganized and unsafe. He was happy that she wouldn't have to endure the assault of noise from the public men's bathrooms. All those urinals out in the open. Combined with the stall doors slamming and the flushing. He usually took care of business as quickly as he could and then practically <u>ran</u> out. The advent of family bathrooms had felt like a gift from above for Luke. He hoped that when they did formal potty training, he could find those individual bathrooms that were starting to crop up in public places.

Luke took over redecoration for sensory processing eagerly, using his set designer background to make it look terrific on a budget. By removing everything that wasn't nailed in or screwed down, he got a chance to see how many things in the bathroom had been distracting Bella when she was taken to the toilet on a schedule. He swapped out the current towels for plain towels in the same color as the walls. Everything that did not need to be on counters was put away. The soap dispenser was now plastic (less breakable) and the medicine cabinet doors were securely fastened so that she couldn't open them. At least, she couldn't do that yet. She was so much more focused now when he brought her in to pee. She paid attention to his gestures to go through the steps to pull down her pants and then her disposable training pants. She sat without getting up every 30 seconds. It was amazing!

Visual modifications can improve a child's focus and limit the temptation to touch or talk about items that they don't need for toileting. Lighting can be less harsh with the use of lower wattage bulbs, warmer bulbs, or dimmer switches. Towels in a solid color, without embellishment, are less stimulating. There are many things that trigger sensory reactions through touch. Sensitive kids may find a line-dried towel too scratchy. They might feel the same way about cheap toilet paper. No one else in their home thinks using either of these items is uncomfortable. Some less-sensitive people don't even realize that the line-dried towels feel all that different from the ones that come out of the dryer. Padded seats can make a huge difference for some kids. When adults are helping to change or wipe a child, the most useful recommendations on modifying touch are to understand that firm pressure is less neurologically activating than light touch, and touch that stays in one spot is less activating than moving touch. A third, but more complicated-to-implement strategy is to use 2 points of touch. For example, wiping a child with one hand while steadying their hip with the other is less activating to the brain than having them lean forward but only have one point of contact on their body; the wipe.

The most effective method to identify what objects and actions affect performance is to remove them one at a time, then observe the resulting changes. Consistent improvement in attention, sensory tolerance, communication, and coordination indicates that an adaptation has had an impact.

Henry was doing well using Corey's larger full bathroom for pre-training. The clutter that was usually scattered on the counter had been relegated to a couple of baskets and shoved into the cabinet. The dimmer switch he installed reduced the lighting glare but still allowed Corey and Henry to see in the room. The only towel out was plain blue, Henry's favorite color. There was no question which towel he should use to dry his hands. The musical timer had been tried and tossed; the shrill sound echoing in the room had made Henry edgier. The padded seat insert with the handles had been a winner. Corey could warm it up with a microwav-

able neck pillow when they were doing their sitting practice, and Henry wanted to sit on it because it was so cozy!

Some children continue to need to use sensory modulation techniques and environmental adaptations in the bathroom long after formal toilet training concludes. <u>This should not be considered a training failure.</u> Success is measured in the degree of independence in all environments with a minimum of effort and time. The child that can use the bathroom in an unfamiliar location without adult assistance by using a few simple sensory-based strategies is still an amazing success!

Chapter 8

Teaching Dressing Skills That Build Independence

Toileting independence is more than eliminating into the potty. Far more. One of the skills essential for using the toilet is the ability to manage clothing. Clothes must be handled correctly to avoid being soiled or soaked. When a child is being diapered, only the adult is paying attention to clothing management. While accidental soiling or soaking could happen during a diaper change, even this event is usually of no consequence to the passively diapered child. Once formal toilet training begins, the child will be the one paying attention to their clothes in important and complex ways.

This isn't always initially clear to a child. It may not be explicitly stated by the adults doing toilet training. Some training approaches give them little practice or boost understanding of this new stage of development. An example would be the use of the standard "potty intensive" or "boot camp" approach. For this training approach, parents and caregivers dress a child in as little clothing as possible. This makes frequent trips to the potty quick and uncomplicated. They are nearly or completely naked during these all-day affairs.

While being undressed makes sense during an intensive training period, it isn't real life. Children need to be able to manage their clothing to be truly independent in toileting. This exceeds the level of skill needed for undressing to climb into the bathtub; they are not removing their clothes to use the potty. Garments are carefully adjusted and adjusted specifically for elimination. Whether dropped too low or lifted to high, incorrect clothing management creates more work to use the toilet, slows down the process, and can be unsafe.

Being able to manipulate clothing efficiently isn't enough. Anyone who has worn Spanx under a formal gown or ski overalls on a ski trip knows that clothing style and fabric choice could make the difference between an accident and a close call. Picking the right garments for toilet training can make the difference between frustration and confident independence.

Sean was doing his second load of laundry…this morning. The first one was wet sheets from Bella's bed, and the second was a combo of her pajamas and the clothes Luke put her in when he got her ready for her day. This should have been no surprise to Sean; Luke loved to dress her in the clothes Maggie bought for her. Both Maggie and Luke liked to see Bella in long dresses with lots of embellishment, worn over a pair of colorful leggings. They thought she looked adorable. They were right about that. She was seriously cute!
Maggie still thought of Bella as a little doll she could dress up. Seeing her look so adorable appeared to help Maggie emotionally handle the fact that Bella had such significant delays in her speech and coordination. Some days it appeared that Luke felt the same way. Or perhaps it was that as a set designer, Luke couldn't resist the chance to play auteur with color and texture with Bella as the "set".

The problem with these outfits was their impracticality for potty training. It was almost impossible for anyone, including Sean, to get Bella undressed enough to get on the toilet before she had an accident. Even if she told them that she needed to go to the bathroom in time, all that fabric and the tight leggings were a nightmare as she wriggled with the need to pee. So here he was, washing her soggy outfit. Right down to the socks and sneakers. At least Sean could now put her in sandals, shorts, and a belly tee. Clothes that made it easier, not harder. Since Luke was out shopping with Maggie, he would be able to get Bella to the toilet in time to prevent an accident before noon. "I really have to speak with him tonight about this", thought Sean. Exactly what to say without offending his husband was the problem.

Choosing Clothes for Pre-Training Success

Three components of garment design make dressing easier during potty training: garment style, fabric choice, and fasteners. Certain features create more challenges, and some choices make life easier for children and adults. Because personal preferences and a family's religion or culture also contribute to clothing selection, every family will make decisions based on a combination of factors. In addition, finances can be an issue for some families. Borrowing clothing or using second-hand stores or tag sales to find lightly worn children's clothing are two affordable ways to find the right clothing on a budget. There may be special events that demand the child wear clothing that they cannot handle in the bathroom without adult assistance. This is understandable and should not create an interruption in pre-training when other pre-training techniques continue to be used on the special day. Overall, pants and shorts are less complicated to manage during toilet training than dresses and skirts. Good pant and short styles have a moderately thick elastic waistband that is easier for kids to locate and grip securely. This eliminates fasteners and improves a child's ability to grasp the waistband to pull the pants up or down when a child urgently needs to use the toilet. Shirts should end at the child's waist, without tails or trim that hangs down. Sleeves that are no longer than ¾ length do not get as wet when hands are being washed. A waist length short-sleeved top is ideal.

Dressing a child in fabrics that minimize the impact of their sensory processing and coordination issues maximizes their success. The worst fabrics to wear for toilet training are silky fabrics that slide around and slip down, and clinging fabrics with a high percentage of Lycra. Rolling their shirt up can improve both skill and safety. But a shirt must stay there to be helpful. A slightly stretchy cotton or cotton blend garment has a slightly "grippy" texture that is more likely to stay rolled up. With a small amount of lycra, a shirt will stay put after it is rolled up and out of the way. Cotton or cotton-blend shorts or pants won't slide down to a child's ankles as easily as a silkier fabric like polyester. Children need to see, feel, and reach the waistband of their underwear, shorts, or pants to pull them up and down. It is also important that they can see their genital area clearly for wiping or directing their urine stream. Limiting how far a child needs to bend forward while balancing on a footstool or in a small space prevents accidents.

It is common for standard "potty intensive" training to suggest that kids are barefoot. Why? Accidents won't always miss their shoes! Hypotonic kids with significant balance and stability issues may need to wear shoes into the bathroom for safe transfers and walking. If they can wear washable shoes or sandals, life is a lot easier for everyone. A second pair of shoes may need to be kept at school if toilet training is happening there as well as at home.

Kids in pre-training may not have the visual-motor skills to use those zippers buttons, snaps, and ties in time to avoid accidents. Even if a child can unzip their jacket independently, they may not have the ability to manipulate the tiny zipper pull commonly used on a pair of jeans. Dressing a child in clothing with fasteners isn't recommended until formal toilet training is very far advanced. Some fasteners that appear easy are anything but. The ties from a waist with a drawstring closure open with just a tug. They can also end up in the toilet bowl or caught inside underwear while pulling shorts or pants back up.

Luke really worried about how his mom would take the news that Bella's wardrobe was going to change during toilet training. She absolutely LOVED dressing her granddaughter up. After hearing that he was gay, then getting married to Sean, and not even in a Catholic church, he knew Maggie held tight to thinking of Bella as her personal dress-up doll. Luke felt that this was the one thing he could give her to make her feel like all the other grandmas at her church group. She adored sharing the photos of Bella in cute outfits on her phone. The ladies at church didn't seem to notice, or at least they didn't say anything out loud, about the fact that Bella never looked directly at the camera.

Bella did look absolutely adorable in most of her clothes. Luke truly enjoyed shopping with his mom for her outfits. He was totally into fashion; always had been. Luke had been simply thrilled during their surrogate's ultrasound appointment when the tech revealed they were having a girl. His mind had immediately gone from "ultrasound picture" to "wedding gown". He had spent the drive home with Sean daydreaming. In his head, he had been lining up one of his friends to design the dress. He might have been married in a tux, but the part of him that loved fashion was going to be able to live vicariously through his daughter.

Nobody was going to like telling Maggie that Bella would be more successful in the bathroom by wearing a short tee and a pair of elastic-waist shorts for the next few months. Maybe for the next few years. Maybe Sean would be willing to tell her. Maybe she would go out and find the cutest little belly tops in the world. Maybe.

Easiest clothing for potty training:
- Cotton or cotton-blend shorts or pants with thick elastic waistbands
- Waist-length cotton short sleeved shirts
- Washable shoes or sandals
- Short cotton-Lycra skirts that can be rolled up

Most challenging clothing for potty training:

- Shirts or tunics or ruffles or shark-bite hems
- Tight leggings with thin waistbands
- Tiny fasteners such as snaps or eye hooks
- Shirts with fringe or beaded bottom edges
- Multiple layers of cloth in separate garments or in the same garment
- Belts and hooks with complicated clasps

What about underwear?

It is time to think about underwear. Some kids at the advanced level of potty training, when they are trained but still need to run to the toilet, do better with no underwear at all. They "go commando"! Fewer layers to manipulate reduce the delays and frustration when garments stick to each other or become bundled together. Some kids, in the midst of formal training, are completely nude. They are usually outdoors, or in areas without floor coverings or upholstered furniture.

Most parents want their kids to wear some form of underwear inside and outside of their home. The type of underwear can be the same in every environment, or it can vary with the circumstance. This "mix-and-match" approach isn't always successful for every child. Children can struggle with code-switching in clothing choice as much as they do with different rules for communication or behavior at home versus at school. This makes it particularly important to understand and explain the potential effects of each clothing choice, and to work on raising frustration tolerance in general.

To move forward as a child approaches full independent toilet use, kids that have been using diapers need to transition to cloth training pants, disposable training pants, or underwear. Each choice has benefits and drawbacks. All three may be used in different locations or used sequentially as toilet training progresses. Adding waterproof liners over underwear or cloth training pants adds a fourth option. When the adults making the decisions about dressing understand more about the impacts of each of these choices, they can take actions that optimize a child's success.

Disposable training pants are the most common choice. Some of this is because of effective marketing. Manufacturers call them "Pull-Ups" or give them another name. Disposable training pants offer very high absorbability, a secure fit, no adhesive diaper tabs, and cute graphics. The manufacturers suggest that a child will see themselves as more grown up.

This is a fallacy. Every child knows that these are a different form of diaper.

A disposable training pant seals up the products of elimination, regardless of where a child is and what they are doing. They can't have the same kind of experience when they have an accident in a disposable training pant that they will in any other underwear choice. And this is when everyone knows that, in reality, this is simply a diaper that the child can slide on and off. They may have a grandparent that wears one. Those are diapers too, with the same powerful and successful marketing strategies to conceal what they really do. Unfortunately, the space-age technology that keeps a child's skin dry and contains the smell can be their worst enemy during potty training. Any urine accident is wicked away before it registers. A bowel accident is barely felt or smelled. Kids that have issues with sensory awareness may never know that they have had an accident at all. These pull-on diapers rarely leak, so kids can keep on playing during and after they pee or poop. This encourages children who are doing something more enjoyable to ignore any urgency sense. They certainly will not tell an adult that they have had an accident. That would mean stopping the fun!

Tiffany was on the fence about using disposable training pants. She preferred the idea of cotton training pants with a waterproof liner, but James's preschool wasn't enthusiastic about them. Neither was Corey. They wanted her to buy disposable training pants because they could be…disposed of, not bagged and sent home. The teachers were fairly convincing, but it seemed so bad for the environment. Corey didn't want to bother with soggy pants either.

Tiffany was convinced that James would be more uncomfortable if he had an accident he could feel. He was well known for not responding when he stepped on a LEGO or when he had food dripping down his chin. She figured that feeling wet pants would move potty training along faster. And she really cared about the environment. All that plastic. If the guilt from thinking that she caused James's issues wasn't bad enough, she knew full well that every diaper in the landfill was adding to stress on Mother Earth.

Don't get me wrong; there are situations in which disposable training pants are necessary and helpful. Many schools do not have the staff to clean up and change a child, particularly an older child, who has repeated accidents while wearing cloth training underwear. Attendance in these programs may be dependent on the use of disposable training pants. Not every family member or friend is as understanding as they could be when a special needs child has a training accident. Accidents on a relative's or a friend's upholstery can mean a difficult end to a holiday celebration. This can be embarrassing for the families as well as the child. Some children are mortified when they are visibly soiled or wet. They would refuse to participate in school, therapy in a clinic, and social events without wearing a disposable training pant.

Alternatives to disposable training pants

One practical adaptation for children with sensory registration or behavioral avoidance issues is to have a child wear a pair of cotton underwear, then add the disposable pants as a second layer. The mess is contained, but the child will have more of a sensory experience of being soiled or wet. Kids will feel it the moment that they urinate as wetness, and this helps them connect the preceding sense of pressure in their bladder and lower abdomen as elimination urgency. Outer clothing needs to be loose enough to accommodate this additional layer. Because disposable training pants are not as bulky as a diaper, this is usually successful. Most children will urinate frequently during the day. This means that a change of training pants has to be available, as well as a way to store wet garments if away from home.

Cloth training pants worn with and without a waterproof liner can be occasionally found at a big box store and are also available online. Families committed to reduce waste and use natural products use them successfully with their typically developing children. The liners and pants aren't imprinted with fun branded characters, but color choice is available. Cotton training pants are made with a thicker crotch layer that absorbs a small degree of leakage. This is helpful for children reaching full toileting independence that may still not always make it to the potty in time to fully avoid an accident. Some kids that are fully trained feel more protected (and thus more confident) by wearing two layers of cloth training underpants or two layers of regular underwear when away from home.

Waterproof liners have elastic leg openings and an elastic waist. They do not fit as smoothly as disposable training pants. This means that tight-fitting clothing may not fit well when using a waterproof liner over training underwear. This can be distressing to a child whose wardrobe hasn't been altered in pre-training. They don't like being uncomfortable or being unable to wear familiar clothing. Very active children may have more leaks while wearing training underwear and liners than they would when wearing disposable pants. Preventing leaks requires a good fit and some attention to help a child get to the bathroom in time to catch small leaks before they become big floods. Changing underwear and liners (and sometimes pants) will increase the amount of laundry that piles up.

Tiffany decided that she would use both cloth training pants as well as disposable pants. She didn't want to alienate the staff at his preschool, and she realized that Dawn probably would think her desire to use cotton pants was too "crunchy granola". She would use them at home when she was in charge of James' care, and simply focus harder on the sensory exercises that his OT had shown her. Tiffany would do her best to get James to move quickly to two layers of cloth pants with her. If she could demonstrate to Corey that James could accomplish a series of dry days, then he might come over to her way of thinking and talk up the idea of cloth pants with Dawn.

Selecting potty training clothes changes with training stages

Pre-training and formal training clothing choices might depend on whether a progressive training or a "potty intensive" approach will used. The intensive strategy often allows the child to be nude from the waist down or to wear elasticized shorts without underwear. They will be spending most of their time in or near the bathroom, consuming liquids frequently and in large enough quantity to require frequent urination.

As the "potty intensive" advances, a child will wear shorts more frequently than staying nude. They make the move to underwear and outer garments when they can manage them in time to prevent accidents. They finally progress to wearing disposable training pants or cotton training pants with a waterproof liner only at night, or when in environments in which they will not have easy access to a toilet. Kids being trained using this approach won't be wearing a wide variety of clothing, and their favorite shorts might end up in the wash every day. They must be able to tolerate changing clothes when it gets soiled, and only wearing the types of clothing that are easy to get up and down quickly. Any irritation from fabrics or clothing style will be magnified in a "potty intensive" because of frequent urination.

With the progressive training approach, there is more flexibility with clothing choices. It may begin as weekend practice in the nude or almost-nude, resembling the "boot camp intensive". Training may start out slowly, with training pants combined with a waterproof liner only when a child is at home. Disposable training pants are worn in other situations. This progresses to wearing a double layer of cotton training pants, and finally progressing to standard underwear during the day, and either a disposable pant or a training pant with a waterproof liner at night.

Cathy Collyer, OTR, LMT

How to teach dressing skills in pre-training

In pre-training, parents and caregivers move away from dressing a passive child to collaborative diapering and dressing to building dressing skills. A child who has successfully completed pre-training is now automatically trying to dress and undress during toileting. Before teaching dressing skills, adults should start paying attention to their own clothing manipulation while using the bathroom. They will realize that they are performing a series of carefully graded movements. Once adults are aware of their own actions, it is easier to appreciate the complexity involved in teaching this skill. This builds both empathy and creativity.

Teaching clothing management for toileting is done in phases. This avoids overwhelming a hypotonic kid who is learning many interconnected skills all at the same time. Asking a child who is brand new to potty training to pull down their pants correctly when they are barely able to recognize the signals of elimination urgency is unrealistic and can lead to accidents. Fully independent clothing management will evolve as a child moves from pre-training to formal toilet training.

The first step is to increase the child's participation in diapering as in Collaborative Diapering. The next step is to build participation in situations where they are strongly motivated to get dressed or undressed. An example would be requiring a child to help remove their clothing so that they can get into the bathtub. Another would be placing their arms into jacket sleeves to go out to play.

Some kids need lots of practice. This can be done by using the "work clothes" strategy. Offer a fun experience (trip to the park, new game, cooking project) which is only obtained by changing to another set of clothing before the fun, and then changing back into their original clothes. The outfit required for the fun to begin is their "work clothes". This prevents the frustration of engaging a child in seemingly useless practice. Most kids balk at taking off their clothing and then putting the same garments right back on. Changing clothes for a short period gets a much better reaction.

Luke made up a simple sticker chart for Bella. Since she couldn't read, he used the PECS pictures the speech therapist had sent in an email attachment. Bella was familiar with some of them, but the drawings of panties, pants, and flushing the toilet were new to her. He got her some llama stickers because that was her new obsession. She couldn't even say the "L" sound, but she was "all llama, all the time" these days. Sima the OT had practiced raising and lowering pants in recent therapy sessions. She suggested they buy a larger size of elastic-waisted pants to make it easier to slide them over the disposable training pants. Sean had gone online searching for llama training pants, and they were a complete hit. Bella didn't want to cover them up with anything else though, so they wouldn't re-order those until summer.

He thought she would be confused about why she was changing her clothes in the middle of the day without having an accident, but Sima suggested that they could tell her that she needed "work clothes" for therapy appointments. This gave them 4 extra clothing changes in both directions: changing before AND after a therapy appointment.

When a child needs to feel successful but isn't going to learn to dress quickly, the "backward chaining" technique can make them experience completion with less frustration. Adults start with teaching the last steps of a task, not the beginning steps. By being active during the last step or two, a child feels they have finished something. When they stop working and an adult takes over, they feel that the adult has been the one who was really in control and involved.

Another frustration-reduction method is to teach children how to pull their pants up before teaching them how to push them down. Pulling pants up is a less graded motor action than partially pushing clothing down. Demonstrate or assist that the waistband is pulled slightly away from the body as it rises over the hips, clearing their genitals and/or underwear. When a child has eliminated into the toilet, there is less time pressure on them. If needed, they can repeat the steps of pulling their pants up without risking an accident. Asking kids to begin pulling up their underpants/pants from the front allows them to see the waistband they are holding while moving the waistband down. The adult initially assists them with bringing the pants up over their buttocks or training diaper, making the action smoother and faster. As a child builds control and speed, adults offer less and less assistance. They begin to teach them to pull up the sides of their waistband after the front is partially raised. Finally, the adult teaches the child to reach behind their body and raise the waistband over their buttocks or underwear. Because a child cannot see the fabric behind them, they need to have developed sufficient motor and sensory skills to complete this step. It isn't expected that a child will be able to smooth out their clothing in pre-training. It is a formal toilet training skill.

Teaching a child to push their pants down is initially done with assistance from an adult. Children often try to pull on their pant leg or a leg band on their underwear to lower their pants. This is easy to understand; they can see and grasp the fabric there easily. The adult stretches the waistband away from the child's abdomen and places the child's fingers on the waistband. As the child pushes their pants down, the adult brings the pants down over the back of their hips. Children need to pull down their pants below their knees, but not to their ankles. Adequate lowering of pants and underpants prevents the accidental soiling of clothes. It also allows a girl's knees to be spread a bit wider apart to accurately wipe after urination.

Hypotonic kids wearing skirts should be initially assisted to tuck their skirt into the waistband of the garment if possible. Dresses are more complicated; they often can be rolled up, possibly under the arms of the child or tucked into a lower neckline. There are some cultures in which young girls are expected to wear dresses or skirts exclusively. Selecting a style and a fabric for dresses during pre-training that will be easier to tuck in or roll up in this manner facilitates training and leads to fewer accidental soiling episodes. Clothing selection and management for the child with low muscle tone can be completely misunderstood and underappreciated as an important skill. The family that takes this seriously and teaches a child well has been both smart and kind. Children want to succeed but cannot be expected to identify what skills and equipment help them the most.

Chapter 9

Building Motivation and Using Incentives That Work

Teaching child with low muscle tone to use the toilet is, at its heart, still teaching a skill. Basic teaching principles will apply:

- *Instruction should be tailored to the individual.*

- *The goal of each step should be understood by the student.*

- *Praise and other incentives for continued effort should be designed with the student's values and needs in mind.*

- *Incentives for participation in learning eventually fade as the student independently uses the knowledge in daily life.*

- *Mistakes during learning must be anticipated and addressed promptly without crushing a student's motivation.*

Kids with hypotonia <u>can</u> learn how to use the toilet. They generally do not start out <u>wanting</u> to learn this skill. They might be fine picking out colorful underpants, or they might like to touch toilet paper or water. No one should misinterpret a desire to play with the water in the potty with wanting to sit on it to poop! It can be difficult to motivate a child to participate in toilet training when, in their mind, using the potty is both unnecessary and frustrating. Wearing a diaper, on the other hand, is familiar and easy. The best teaching skills for potty training must be combined with the strongest incentives for learning and practicing a complex sensory-motor skill.

What to say, and how to say it for best effect

Every child learns best and performs best when the instructions are a match for their current attention and communication skills. Children that take a long time to process spoken language but respond well to signing, graphics, or gestures need the adults doing training to use those non-verbal strategies in teaching. If attention or memory are limited, they need to have routines and receive cues that make paying attention and recalling information easier. Repetition is almost always necessary to establish new learning into habitual behavior.

Every teaching moment begins with getting the student's attention. When kids have been passively diapered for years, initially bringing their attention to peeing and pooping might take some effort. Kids who have already experienced the shift to "collaborative diapering", as described in chapter 4, are primed to know what they are doing and to pay more attention when directed to sit on the toilet.

Children who have done collaborative diapering at the beginning of pre-training learned the words for body parts and the products of elimination. They are familiar with single-step instructions during diapering. The words, graphics, signs, and gestures that were successfully learned in collaborative diapering can be recycled for use during pre-training and in formal training. These words could be as simple as "more", "done", and "up" or "down".

Using photos and graphics

Not all kids need photos and graphics to help them learn how to use the toilet. But when they do, they can move learning forward quickly. Many teachers and psychologists recommend the use of graphic images to help kids learn the steps for using the toilet. The images can depict a person performing each action, or they can represent only the equipment. Kids learn that a 2-dimensional image represents a live action. PECS are a common system of graphic images familiar to many therapists and teachers. They are available online from companies that sell materials for special education. The details in the individual images range from very simple to complex. Parents and professionals can also make their own images, including photos of the child using the toilet.

An example of the use of a photo or a full graphic would be a still image of a person washing their hands. The abbreviated graphic would be a drawing of hands under a faucet, with soap bubbles surrounding the hands. Both are describing the action the child needs to perform: washing their hands after they use the toilet. Stringing together a sequence of images on a large poster can guide a child through each step, all the way up to drying their hands and leaving the bathroom. When used in pre-training or formal toilet training, these posters are mounted in the diaper changing area or in the bathroom. The graphics or photos can become movable objects when they are laminated and backed with Velcro. A child either places the image on a chart to begin the step on the laminated card, or they remove the card from a previously full poster after completion of that step.

The use of graphics can also be helpful to increase a child's attention during toilet use and used as a motivator to sustain participation. Many children enjoy the physical act of moving Velcro-backed pictures. This physical action helps them define the beginning or ending of a task, making it easier for them to advance through the many steps involved in using the bathroom. While PECS and other images can be used only during toilet training, they have a more powerful effect on behavior when they are used in other situations at home or in school.

Overall, the decision to use images to teach toileting should be made by identifying the benefits and the limitations for the child and either for the teachers (if done at school) or the caregivers at home. Kids need to be able to connect the idea that a 2-dimensional image represents a live action. Kids who are familiar with the concept that a 2-dimensional image represents a live action.

A child's entire team can provide input on the decision to use graphics and to build a vocabulary around toileting. Any system that spans locations requires coordination. If communication is sketchy, this would make pivoting and flexing as a child gains skills more difficult. There are children who are so familiar with PECS and other symbolic communication strategies that it would be much more difficult to do potty training without using them! There are other children that have never been exposed to this technique or who find images more interesting than a live model. Distraction is never a good choice! Because complex physical skills are harder to display in an image, there are situations in which graphic images cannot capture details well enough to be the primary teaching tool at advanced levels. Some teams start with PECS and switch to verbal and signed directions when a child is in the final stages of toilet training.

Lewis looked at the sticker chart Jordan brought over when she dropped Henry off for his weekend. It looked like someone had gone nuts in the arts and crafts section of Walmart. There wasn't an inch that wasn't covered in bright colors, photo collages, and messages of encouragement. All for a kid who didn't recognize the letters in his name or respond when his name was called! Lewis thought this would be a waste of his precious time with Henry this weekend.
Lewis knew he had no choice but to go along with it. Refusing to sign on would be an immediate argument. But he didn't see the point. Henry had never been successful with a sticker chart before. Colorful or plain. He had managed to master the token system at school: he got a fake penny to drop into the piggy bank when he followed steps of his routine.
Lewis suspected that Henry's teachers and therapists were the architects of the latest attempt to use a sticker chart home. They were great at teaching him other things, warm and caring even when Henry had a meltdown. Without a new angle on using stickers to celebrate peeing, Lewis wasn't sure this time was going to be any different from the last one.

He found out that Henry could and did use the chart. It was a hit! Henry understood that he only got a sticker when he peed into the potty. He expected it right away, so Lewis started storing them in a baggie on a bathroom shelf.

Kids that are motivated by tokens or star charts should regularly reminded of them during training. The concept of using incentives or rewards can be initially distasteful to some parents. It is easy to appreciate their concerns that their child's cooperation is to be expected, not "bought". Having a tangible, and visible, reward does seem to be helpful for many kids and adults. Paychecks and online reviews come to mind. One reason Dr. Harvey Karp's Happiest Toddler on the Block communication techniques work extremely well is because they build cooperation with negotiation and compassion, not bribes. While every adult uses some form of praise during training, there are kids who aren't the least bit impressed with in a bathroom song-and-dance. They give it the fisheye or worse. "Know your audience" is the lesson if that is the response received from making a big fuss over potty training success! Some kids absolutely insist on a tangible reward for their efforts. Verbal praise doesn't register as an incentive for them. Incentives do not have to be stickers or foods. Many older children want their reward in the form of an experience, like time at the park or the ability to control what is for dinner tomorrow night. It is common for parents to worry that their children will someday refuse to use the toilet unless they receive candy or get a new toy at the end of week. This is a realistic concern. The solution is to fade rewards gradually and ramp up expectations for full participation without "payment" in the other areas of a child's life.

Choosing incentives that work

Making a solid incentive plan is far more complicated than asking a child what they want as a reward. Screen time and candy often are high on every child's list. A child's requested motivators may not be the ones that parents or caregivers are willing or able to use. It might not even be effective to use the motivators that a child suggests. For example, screen time isn't available or allowed in most educational programs, and some families wish to heavily restrict their child's access to screens of all kinds. Sugary foods or salty snack foods could interfere with a child's diet and even their health.
Access to specific snacks or shows can be inconsistent or completely unavailable. This interruption leads to a disruption in their faith in a meaningful reward system. Selecting incentives for success that are more widely available across all training environments is strongly recommended for kids that can't handle choosing between a small number of rewards or having to wait to receive one. Incentives at the beginning of training need to be small enough to be repeated frequently throughout the day and in the weeks to come. Large rewards can't be delivered multiple times a day. When a large or expensive reward fails to be motivating, there is no space to increase this incentive. Early incentives also need to be delivered immediately for children to mentally

connect their actions with receiving a reward.

The most successful motivations and rewards are meaningful to the child, easy to deliver, small in size, and can be provided soon after successful goal accomplishment. It is entirely possible that a hug or a "high-5" would be a free, healthy, readily available, and totally successful reward.

A simple star chart is a common way to offer and record incentives. The opportunity to earn stars, with their motivating rewards, must be relatively frequent throughout the day. The chart is visible in their home, but it could also be portable so that school staff can use it during the day. The selected in-centive needs to be concrete and initially able to be delivered immediately to teach the connection between actions and rewards. Emphasizing the positive is important; there should be no sense that accidents or refusals are punished by not getting a star. There will always be another chance to earn a star in the future.

The "stars" may need to be themed stickers that have meaning to the child. For every child that likes actual stars, there are kids that want car stickers or Elsa stickers. Again, knowing the child helps adults select the right tools for the job. Stars for a standard chart usually accumulate to be exchanged for a reward. The child now must wait for that reward to be delivered. If a child has never used a star chart before, trialing their ability to use this system can be first used with a task that they have already mastered or partially mastered. This trial chart can be as simple as a few hand-drawn boxes on a piece of paper. For example, if they occasionally put their empty cup or plate into the sink, this becomes the action that earns a star for their chart. They or their teacher, parent or therapist either places their star on the chart right after they deposit their cup, or they observe an adult doing so while the adult describes what they are doing and why. The reward to delivered right after the star goes up on the chart. Because novel routines can be rejected due only to the changed routine, adults need to have patience and use as much testing time as needed to determine that a child understands the relationship between their actions and how they earned a star and a concrete reward.

One of the most common questions parents and caregivers have regarding the use of incentives is "Do I reward him for a tiny amount of urine?" In general, the answer is "yes", particularly at the beginning of training, or with a child that immediately interprets any withholding of rewards as either punishment or rejection. Hypotonic kids frequently need more help to figure out what they are supposed to be doing. They might not be sure that peeing is the goal right away! Until the adult is certain that the child is intentionally withholding urine or feces, they should be given the benefit of the doubt and provided with the agreed-upon reward.

One common toilet training approach includes asking a child to sit on the toilet without knowing if they have any urinary or bowel urgency, or even knowing if they have enough urine or feces present for elimination. Some kids will have just eliminated into their training pants. They could be constipated. If the child is cooperative but is unable to eliminate, this can be confusing and frustrating for them. They will not receive their reward unless the goal was <u>sustained sitting</u> rather than elimination.

Shaming a child after soiling or wetting their clothes is not helpful. Ignoring the mess in a child's pants, accidental or intentional, is also a missed opportunity. The most helpful response is to tell a child that they didn't succeed with getting their incentive at that moment. They will get another chance soon today. Maybe very soon. And figure out what went wrong as quickly as possible. Then the real work begins; the child needs to be involved in cleaning themselves and redressing. This means there is no opportunity to play or watch a show on the large screen TV in the living room across from the bathroom. They help toss out disposable pants or place their soiled garments in the correct location (if this can be done safely), and obtain all of the needed wipes and clean clothing. Expectations and consequences for ignoring an adult's instructions might be reviewed. All of this is done while still being positive about being independent and firm about consequences for defense.

Sean was so excited to start getting Bella involved in her own diapering. He had been lobbying quietly for this for years, but Luke was so resistant. Sean decided that because she was non-verbal and had so many delays that it was going to be hard anyway, and he let it go. But now the OT was pushing both of them harder to have Bella always get a fresh diaper and wipes, even to try wiping herself! The idea of her wiping her body after a bowel movement made Sean a bit nauseous, to be honest. He imagined how badly it could go and wanted to order some of those

PPE gowns he saw nurses wearing in the ICU. One of them in the bathroom shouldn't be decorated in feces during the process!!

He was impressed with how well she managed wiping after peeing. It gave him hope that she could eventually wipe her body after pooping. For now, he wiped her first after pooping and she did some cursory wiping when he finished. It wasn't perfect, but she was participating and she knew what to do.

Moving on from rewards

Corey had always found disciplining James nearly impossible. He depended on Tiffany to rescue both him and James when things went south. James knew this, so he seemed to wait until his mom stepped away to let some of his fits really rip. At least, that is how it appeared to Corey. He did not have a poker face, and so it was obvious when he was frustrated or angry. Just when it would have been better to walk away, Corey found himself telling James to stop doing something, or start doing something, or to be quiet.

Successful potty training requires that a child isn't rewarded forever for independently using the toilet. Ending incentives is necessary. Research on incentive programs in general has indicated that when a person is motivated exclusively by rewards, their behavior doesn't improve over the long term. Star charts and reward systems morph into expectations for independence. This is the exit plan, and every potty training plan needs one.

There are two effective strategies for getting rid of incentives: polite ignoring and fading rewards. "Fading" in this situation means extending the period before a reward is earned until there is no longer a reward at all. The type of incentives used later in potty training, when the goal is to remain continent all day or continent for several days at a time, can be both larger, less concrete than a snack or toy, with a delay between accomplishment and receiving the reward. A trip to the car wash as a reward for a week of successful potty use during the day can be exciting. Some car wash sites have a viewing section where children can watch the cars as they get scrubbed and rinsed. Others allow the car's occupants to remain in their car as it moves through the soap and water. This could be absolute heaven for a child!

"Polite ignoring" is the term Dr. Harvey Karp uses when adults do not attend to minor behavioral infractions in toddlers. It can be used it in a slightly more sophisticated manner during toilet training. An adult acknowledges the child's request for a reward in an extremely flat and brief manner. This communicates that the adult is less interested in delivering rewards without totally ignoring a child. The conversation is switched the subject to something far more fun and exciting. Even better? Change of venue. In law, a change of venue is where a trial is held in a different location than the town or county in which the crime was committed. The decision is made that the accused will get a fairer trial outside of town. For toilet training, moving a child away from the familiar site of delivering the reward can help a child separate the action of using the toilet from the expectation of an incentive. Polite ignoring combined with a change in venue can be a useful combination to fade the expectation of a reward.

If a child won't shift their attention, or if they become agitated, this is a chance to use another excellent Happiest Toddler technique: patience stretching. Using patience stretching doesn't accomplish the goal of eliminating incentives. It builds a child's frustration tolerance and prepares them emotionally for the incentives to end. With patience stretching, they will get their reward, but they will have to wait while the adult engages in something else for a very short time.

Tiffany decided that Dr. Karp's Patience Stretching was so successful she was going to use it on her husband! She had not started it with anything like enthusiasm. While it was explained to her, she thought "This sounds stupid and a waste of time. James screams when he doesn't get what he wants right away." But she decided to try it. The next time he requested juice, she was animated as she eagerly agreed, then held up her hand and said "Oh, I forgot. I need look find a special straw!" and quietly counted out loud to 10. That first time he started the screaming as soon as she walked past the cabinet with the juice boxes. He knew that she wasn't moving as quickly as usual when he said "Joooey", his word for juice. So he screamed it! When Tiffany cheerily replied "You want juice box. Yes, yes, YES! You get juice box" and repeated this twice while wiping the countertop, his wails dropped a few decibels. That was a week ago. Now she could leave the room, flush to toilet in the downstairs bath, and then return to the kitchen while he still

waited patiently. As long as James always got what she had agreed to deliver, she could buy herself about 90 seconds without triggering a fit. This was actually...
working out!

Chapter 10

Selecting A Plan for Success

Finally…it is time to start formal toilet training!

- *What are the anticipated challenges of toilet training?*
- *What strengths does a child have that can be used to make progress?*
- *Which approach is the best overall fit for a child?*
- *Which approach is best for the adults participating in potty training?*

If these questions cannot be at least partially answered before formal training begins, then everyone is facing more stress than they need. Targeted pre-training is designed to fill in the blanks in these questions. This chapter will help explain how to pick a plan that fits well and gives a child with low muscle tone the best chance for success.

Sean and Luke were not in agreement on how to make more progress. This bothered Luke way more than it bothered Sean, because Luke believed that Maggie and Padriac, Sean's parents, would take their son's side, whatever he said. Sean hoped so; Maggie could be loud and convincing when she wanted to be. Padriac would go along with anything his wife said. He believed that giving in was not giving up. That was one of the secrets to a good marriage, as his dad had shared with Sean on his wedding day. Sean didn't like disagreeing with his husband on anything for very long. He had inherited Padriac' distaste for argument. He simply wanted what was best for Bella, and he thought that Luke was wrong on which approach to take in formal toilet training.
Sean wanted to go for the "potty intensive" approach during Christmas vacation.

He felt that Bella would learn more and learn faster if she was repeating the same things for a series of days, and she didn't have school or therapies during that time. She would not have to wear a diaper for those days. Sometimes she held her urine until she had a diaper to pee into. That could make the gradual approach TOO gradual. Take-a-year-or-more gradual!

Luke knew Sean had a point about this. Actually he thought Sean had a few good points. Not that he told his husband about this. And, in truth, he feared what staying near the bathroom with Bella all day, every day, with repeated accidents, would do to him. Those smells, the mess. It would be hard.

Choosing between the "potty intensive" or the gradual approach

Deciding whether to do a "potty intensive/boot camp" or a gradual approach is a decision that some parents make right away. They look at the calendar and figure out that they have one week of vacation from work and school next month. It gets earmarked for intensive training. Other parents have awful memories of the mega-tantrums resulting from interrupting their child from play to take them to the toilet. These parents decide that a "potty intensive" will create more aggravation than they think they could tolerate.

Many parents and professionals aren't sure which way to go, and it can come down to making a pro/con list. The decision is made easier when they identify what constitutes a "full stop" for their child and for them. If there is no way to carve out exclusive time and energy for an intensive approach, or if a child will become frightened by being restricted to a portion of their home while naked and urinating around the clock, then the gradual training approach is probably best. If a child learns best when given intensive training without distraction, then the intensive approach may fit them like a glove.

The approach must fit the adults training as well as the child being trained. Not every adult has the required patience and the intense focus needed to do the "boot camp" approach to potty training. This isn't a criticism of their character. This training strategy initially results in repeated accidents and increasing frustration for everyone. Some adults will only consider an intensive approach: they cannot imagine spending months on training and are willing to devote a short period to nothing else but potty training, provided it really works. They want to see definitive proof of progress within a few days. This keeps <u>their</u> motivation up and they won't be distracted by day-to-day concerns. Being torn in many directions often means nobody gets the attention they need.

Who is going to be starting the training process?

It is often assumed that toilet training will begin at home. There are no protocols or policies, no bad peer models (we hope), and lots of opportunities to try new equipment. Home is where kids spend more time, and no one is as motivated for a child's success in toilet training as their family. This does not always make their home the <u>right</u> place to begin formal training. Parents should not feel ashamed or be self-critical if their child responds well to potty training at school or daycare staff but gives them a very hard time at home. Children tune into the attitudes of the people around them. They perceive confidence, calmness, and enthusiasm without a word being said out loud. And the opposite. Something as simple as an anxious adult's body language during toileting can throw them off.

If potty training gets started at school, everyone at home needs to learn which prompts and what level of assistance are being used successfully. This prevents creating two competing sets of behaviors and expectations for a child to follow. It is possible to do both types of training in different locations. A child can go through intensive training at home during a school break, building some essential skills, without being fully trained. They return to school and continue to use the gradual training approach there, but they now have a greater degree of independence.

Training order: pee first or poop first?

It is common for potty training to be separated. Many times, a child achieves independent use of the toilet for urination apart from toileting independence for bowel movements. This is true for both the intensive approach and the gradual training approach. Children will urinate more frequently each day, giving them more practice in recognizing elimination urgency. Their routines for clothing management, wiping, flushing, and handwashing build skills rapidly as they are done multiple times a day. Other than wiping, these skill transfer from one type of elimination to the other. Accurate wiping is less of a messy experience than wiping after a bowel movement. Urination urgency and elimination is a less intense sensory experience for most kids. It is rarely uncomfortable, and rarely carries with it negative memories in the ways that recalling constipation or intestinal cramping can complicate bowel training.

There are some children who are trained to have bowel movements first, and later learn to urinate in the toilet. This training order is often seen with children that have exposure to "elimination communication". It is also done when a child's bowel movements are easily anticipated; some kid's digestion is so regular that you can set a watch by their bowel movements! Just because starting toilet training by teaching a child to poop is the less common sequence doesn't mean that it is the <u>wrong</u> approach. Deciding to train a child to use the toilet for bowel movements before urination should make sense to the child's entire team, but it absolutely can be the right choice for the right child.

The "potty intensive"

Also known as the "boot camp" method of training, this approach requires that a child will be taken to the potty on a very frequent basis during the daytime to pee. Potty intensives are not done to teach a child to poop. A child will only have one bowel movement per day on average, and some kids have one every other day. The child in "boot camp" spends much of their day close to a toilet, accompanied by an adult that either brings them to the toilet or supervises their use of the potty. Their ability to leave home or roam around the whole house is very limited. The needs of other children and the adult's other responsibilities will take a back seat for the adult doing a training intensive. They aren't doing school pick up and may not even be able to leave sight of the child in training. Someone else is taking on the important things that can't be tackled while helping a child in "boot camp".

Except during naps and bedtime, the adult in charge offers the child frequent liquids throughout the day, then brings the child to the toilet or potty seat to pee. The child is lightly dressed or could be completely undressed from the waist down. They may wear plastic sandals or be barefoot. There are lots of spare clothes, wipes, and washable toys around. Because the risk of accidents goes up when a child isn't wearing a diaper, this limits the location of training to spaces that have non-porous floors, and to seating surfaces that can be disinfected. Sticker charts and incentives or rewards are used throughout the day. At first, the reward is given for sitting promptly when asked. As the "potty intensive" progresses, the bar for rewards is raised. Incentives are still delivered, but they are given for more advanced and independent toileting skills.

The adult running the intensive is patient but also enthusiastic and encouraging. Conversations with the child always circle back to talking about toileting and elimination urgency. Children should successfully urinate in the potty most of the time. But nobody is perfect at timing use, and children can't sit for hours. This means that there will also be accidents. Accidents are anticipated in a training intensive. Not making it to the toilet in time is dealt with calmly and compassionately.

The "potty intensive" approach works better with a child that can:

- leave a toy or other activity without significant hesitation or agitation when told to use the toilet.
- remain standing while removing clothing with minimal assistance, sit comfortably for at least 3-5 minutes on the potty or toilet, and wipe/ flush with minimal assistance or verbal prompting. A child that needs more assistance feels over-handled at the end of a long day of repeated toileting.
- follow instructions and maintain a reasonably calm state while their day is heavily focused on toilet training.
- accept restrictions regarding what access to only part of the house.
- understand and value rewards and incentives.
- handle more frequent potty accidents than they are used to without meltdowns; accidents will happen!

- **Recall routines and remember both new skills and how successful they were when intensive training ends.**

For many children with low muscle tone, this approach tends to be used as either a "finishing line" or a "jump start" event, or both. The child could have worked on all the components of toileting through a gradual approach. They are now ready to put it all together. But it works if you do an intensive beginning as well. Beginning with an intensive approach for a component of toilet training can get training off to a faster start because the intense focus makes it easy to practice many of the pre-training skills together for strong learning in a short period of time.

When a particular part of the toileting routine is difficult for a child to learn, parents and caregivers can use a focused "mini-intensive" to clarify the message. An example would be the child who is struggling with the ability to identify urinary urgency. They are not being defiant; there is little awareness that their bladder is full and they need to pee. Now.

In intensive training, this child is offered a favorite drink very frequently and asked to sit on the potty every 10-15 minutes. They are told what urgency feels like, where it is felt, and as they drink more and more, they are asked to describe any change in sensation. Even if they have an accident, it is reviewed like a "CSI" episode so that they child connects the subtle sensations with elimination urgency. The adult doing the training intensive rewards all efforts sand celebrates successes, then repeats the experience until a stronger connection is made. This routine may only be possible on weekends or extended holidays, but it can quickly propel toilet training independence ahead.

Before deciding to use the "potty intensive" approach, families and caregivers need to decide if this must be altered or extended based on a child's specific needs and challenges. Every hypotonic child is different. Success is not assured and should not be promised. Some children <u>and</u> adults react very poorly to failure or to switching approaches out of frustration. There is no shame in choosing the gradual approach if either the child or the adults doing training would find a training intensive too stressful.

The gradual approach

This is exactly what it sounds like; progressively building a child's ability to complete the steps of toileting. Children progressively move from being assisted for toileting to being independent in all steps of elimination from sensing urgency to flushing and wiping. Using the gradual approach is a continuation and refinement of targeted pre-training.

There are three major differences between pre-training and formal toilet training with a gradual approach:

- In formal toilet training using the gradual approach, the speed with which independence is expected is faster. Kids are not given as much time to "coast" before the next skill is taught and absorbed.

- Multiple skills are taught at the same time. While gradual training may begin with teaching one skill at a time, it doesn't stay that way. By the end of gradual training, children are being taught many skills in a single week. These include timing bathroom trips before going outside to play,

- Caregivers will require independent use of a variety of skills *at the same time and in the right order.* Kids are expected to complete the steps for clothing management and getting on and off the toilet. The child may have to take out the things they need for toileting in advance, such as moving their wipes next to the toilet. A child that was prompted for undressing and hand washing in pre-training will be supervised and given the tools they need for hygiene. They will not necessarily be told <u>what</u> to do and <u>when</u> to do it.

Cathy Collyer, OTR, LMT

The gradual approach works better with kids who:

- **Can handle some inconsistency; they will wear a diaper some of the time, in some situations.**
- **Can afford to learn slowly. If they need to be trained to attend summer camp or be ready for a general education class, they might need a faster approach.**
- **Have a very complicated life that they cannot/won't suspend for the period of time needed for "boot camp". These kids can't miss a week of therapy or will be intensely upset from not attending social or extra-curricular activities.**
- **Become very discouraged, ashamed, or angry when they have accidents. The gradual approach can build skills in a way that should minimize accident frequency.**

How to move a child into underwear

Kids doing either type of potty training eventually have to make the leap from training pants and into underwear. This is one of the biggest transitions that occurs in formal training. It is the hardest transition for many children, and the hardest for many parents and caregivers. Accidents while wearing underwear are more frequent than while wearing a diaper. These accidents are more likely to result in both messes and tears for everyone. Diapers have been the training wheels preventing the emotional and physical consequences of not getting to the toilet in time.

Switching between training pants and underwear within a day is done frequently during toilet training with some kids. It can be difficult for some kids to understand the criteria for when it is OK to wear training pants, and when they need to wear underwear. Making the transition in distinct stages assists the child who likes rules. Buying underwear in a favorite color or

128

printed with cartoon characters they love may make the change to underpants more appealing. But before anyone runs out to find Paw Patrol panties, it is time to understand what else can make this transition easiest to handle. Instead of seeing the chance to move from diapers to underpants as taking a victory lap, the transition into underwear needs to be seen as a demanding period of greater focus and energy. New learning is crystalizing while old routines are being abandoned. Maintaining positivity through a period of more frequent accidents can be difficult. One answer is to "double down" on some of the pre-training magic strategies of routines, incentives, and sensory processing strategies that helped kids transition from passively being diapered to actively participating in toileting.

Incentives might take on more significance in this phase, rather than be faded away. Routines that help kids stay calm usually also help them stay more aware; they need to be calm and responsive to their body's signals to avoid accidents. Kids with continuing sensory processing issues might need a more finely tuned sensory diet. Some parents put two pairs of underwear on their child as back-up protection for accidents during underwear-only training. This means their clothing choices need to accommodate that extra layer. A child who is uncomfortable in tight clothing has been given a good reason to balk at transitioning into underwear.

A child who went through pre-training and still has issues with constipation and diarrhea may not be ready for formal bowel training until they have predictable, pain-free, and formed bowel movements. A child who intention-ally withholds, or intentionally soils or wets, isn't displaying physical inability. They are responding to an emotional issue that might be obvious or one that might be difficult to identify.

Bowel continence is often achieved after urinary continence in almost all kids. Most healthy children have a bowel movement on awakening (i.e. before you hear them roaming around in their room), shortly after a meal, or after being physically active. Once they have had a bowel movement, they will not have another one for many hours, probably not until the next day. Maybe two days; bowel activity doesn't require daily bowel movements to be considered normal by. This means that if a child has a bowel movement in the morning and is also continent of urine during the day (daytime dryness), then they can wear their underwear all day long!

Daytime dryness almost always happens before nighttime dryness. Dryness at home and/or school is usually achieved before dryness in public activities. The first is mostly physiological. Awakening enough to get to the toilet in time while holding urine until they reach the toilet in the middle of the night takes a level of physical maturity. The second is often environmental. Not knowing where the nearest toilet is, being too far from the toilet, and being too distracted to attend to subtle urgency cues all increase the risk of accidents away from home. Illness and changes in routine frequently trigger temporary lapses in continence. This should be anticipated and incorporated into any plan. After 4-8 consecutive days of daytime dryness, it will be time to ask a child in formal toilet training to wear underwear during the day at home for at least a short period of time.

Not all hypotonic kids need this extended period of daytime dryness to make the transition. A longer period of daytime dryness while wearing a diaper is suggested to build everyone's confidence. It can "buy time" to observe consistent toileting skills in a variety of activities and environments. This observation period is done on the days when a child can still be near a bathroom when they need one. Adults are close by and responsive to the child's signals for urgency.

When parents and caregivers are quick to act after an accident (the child has not withheld and "spilled over", or intentionally eliminated in their underwear), and they can do so without shaming a child, they decrease the emotional impact of an accident on a child. Accidents become learning experiences for both adults and children. The adults surrounding the child need to be alert for subtle signs of stress at the dinner table or at bedtime that can be traced back to a series of accidents or a single accident occurring in an important location or situation. The most important teaching point is that greater responsibility for toileting and managing accidents is now shifted onto the child. It can take time for a child that has worn a diaper for years to be fully responsible for using the bathroom. Moving out of training pants is a process rather than a quick transition. Full daytime dryness will not send every training pant or diaper in the trash. As the child develops more nighttime physical maturity, training pants are no longer worn for bed. The child is completely toilet trained!

Jordan and Lewis thought that their family wouldn't survive the "potty intensive" style of training. Simone, Mia's daughter from her first marriage, had made it clear that her teen friends would be "totally grossed out ", in her words, by Henry walking around naked and peeing in potty. Simone said she was sure that her social life would never recover. Simone was also the only sibling that couldn't stay with another parent during an intense training period. Simone had been through a lot, and Jordan was always a bit worried that she wasn't giving her enough attention. She really was a great kid. She simply couldn't make Simone's life harder.

Danielle was sure she could do the intensive training during the day while she was there alone with him. She had weekends off. The nights and weekends that Henry wasn't with Lewis, it would be Jordan's responsibility to do the training intensive. The chance that Jordan, Danielle and Henry could make much progress while the two middle kids were staying at Lewis's for a long holiday weekend seemed unlikely. Sharon was still in Florida, playing Mahjong and getting a nice tan. Jordan thought cynically, "When she comes back up north, she will pass judgement on everyone and everything. That won't add much to the stress." All of Jordan's days lately seemed like that movie "Groundhog Day". She woke up and the routine took off.

Update: Henry managed to do pretty well with the intensive approach. Danielle turned out to have some clear advantages to offer. He listened well to her, and she took no prisoners when he balked. By the time the weekend rolled around, Danielle could explain to Jordan what had worked and what had failed for her. The treat/reward choice was clear and so was the preferred beverage: Yoo Hoo. He peed like a racehorse when he drank her thinned-out cups of chocolate milk through the day.

The gradual approach for children with global developmental delays

Some hypotonic children have profound global developmental delays. This means that they have significantly delayed development in many areas of abilities: cognitive, communication, motor control, sensory processing, and self-care skills. Because of the degree of their delays, professionals often tell their parents that they will not be ready for training any time soon. Children who have significant global delays who use a toileting schedule may stay dry for extended periods, but they rarely react to urinary urgency by independently indicating the need to use the toilet without training. This is incredibly frustrating for their families. They often take the advice of inexperienced professionals and drop all attempts at training.

For these children, this is almost always a mistake.

The risks of long delays before starting toilet training without using targeted pre-training, are clear; every year of being passively diapered reinforces the sense that eliminating in a diaper is what is expected. They develop the habit of ignoring being diapered and what happens "down there" that lead to needing a diaper! The child can connect diapering with singing or play. The adults caring for them may not recognize this play is extending the delay in toilet training. They believe they are building skills during diapering. These satisfying play routines become more and more difficult to alter as time passes. Requesting a sudden increase in participation can bring out fear or agitation in a globally delayed older child. This, in turn, leads parents and caregivers to believe that the child is <u>still</u> not ready to begin any aspect of potty training.

The presence of global developmental delays will require that every new learning task is broken down into manageable parts. The bathroom and the tools of toileting may need to be adapted to increase attention and optimize motor skills. Almost every part of the Collaborative Diapering process is adapted for ease and faster learning. A firm diapering or toileting schedule is developed once their family and caretakers realize when they are most likely to eliminate. A child who has learned their pre-training routine and can reduce accidents with its use is still a success!

Using extended periods of pre-training can help a globally delayed child knit together the subtle physiologic cues of elimination urgency. Because of their delays in communication and motor skills, it might be difficult for adults to interpret their signals that indicate that they know they need to use the toilet. Agitation or self-stimulatory behavior that is observed after meals should be taken as possible indications of elimination urgency. In this way, increasing the globally delayed child's recognition of elimination urgency can be surprisingly quick. One day a child may get herself to the toilet off-schedule, but it may be because she now knows that she needs to "go"!

An excellent reason to build skills in these kids is the fact that when they are active participants in diapering and toileting it discourages sexual predators. These kids will be in special extra-curricular programs and self-contained classes as they grow. An older child that is actively participating signals to a potential predator that they are more capable in this area, including potentially being capable of communicating negative experiences. A predator will decide that this child is not a desirable victim.

Every hard-won gain in any self-care skill improves the profoundly delayed child's cognition, their ability to communicate, and their sensory processing abilities in everyday life. Improving safe transfers on and off the toilet, assisting more with clothing management, with wiping, and with hand washing make their lives better, even if they remain dependent in some other ways. All progress at home should be reported to and recognized by the child's team. The undeniable evidence of learning can have radical effects on a child's life. Their family needs less time and effort for diapering. They can bring their child to more events with more confidence. The child's personal care aides they have now will reconsider how they view a globally delayed child who gains visible skills. So will the child's teachers and therapists. These professionals may decide that a teaching or treatment strategy they considered too advanced for this child is now worth trying!

Chapter 11

Wiping, Flushing, and Washing Hands

Toileting isn't done when the toilet gets filled up. They need to wipe. The potty needs to be flushed. Hands must be washed and wiped. Hygiene is important in the bathroom, and it begins to be more of the child's responsibility in targeted pre-training. By formal training, it is a part of everyday life. Or it should be. If flushing, washing, wiping, and drying hasn't been mastered before formal training begins, the time to build these skills is at the start of formal toilet training.

Kids that have had typical motor development throughout childhood have had many subtle advantages to learn how to master personal hygiene before they are potty trained. They have watched adults use the sink and the bathroom from an early age. They have been able to stand on a footstool to wash and flush, and they have manipulated all types of tissues as well as played with the toilet paper in their home bathrooms. The hypotonic child may have been unable to stand and explore their home in those early years. They may have used a walker that did not allow them to get into the bathroom, or they may have been so heavily supervised and "therapized" that free exploration was limited.

Teaching a child with low muscle tone how to do the essential hygiene tasks needed for independent toileting doesn't mean that they will not need practice and supervision for a while. Complex skills often need both to be fully learned. Well into the preschool years, many typically developing kids need reminders to "finish the job". Teachers often use adult and peer demonstrations and peer pressure to build a student's awareness of the need for hygiene skills at school.

Bella loved water play. She adored the bath, loved aqua therapy, and couldn't wait to play with soap and water when she was told to wash her hands. Bella had to have the water turned off and the soap pump taken out of reach for her to stop water play! Leaving things out and turning your back on Bella risked deco-

rating you so that you were wearing citrus-scented soap in your hair and on your clothes. She was very "generous" that way.

This didn't mean that she had any awareness of her hands being soiled or felt any disgust once she saw feces on her fingers after "exploring" her diaper. Maggie felt her breakfast rise in her throat the first time she saw her granddaughter dip a hand into her diaper. The thought occasionally occurred to Maggie that Bella did it just to get a chance to play with the soap and water in the sink. There was no way to know for sure. Asking her about the reason for this behavior would be pointless. Bella had just mastered a few signs and had no verbal language at all yet.

Hypotonic kids, like all kids, vary in their motivation for hygiene activities. They may be fascinated with using soap and water and enjoy the sound of a flushing toilet in a small, well-tiled bathroom. They might want to play in the water with relish and make a mess, and they may want to flush the toilet repeatedly. Things can also go the other way. They may cringe at washing and flushing, and resist being wiped or wiping their <u>own</u> body after peeing or pooping. Drawn-out hand washing sessions, where everyone and everything gets wet, are common behaviors for the sensory-seeking child. Their parents wonder if greater independence in hygiene is truly a <u>good</u> thing!

Not every challenge with bathroom hygiene comes from a child's sensory processing issues. Some children need to work on their balance or their ability to use both hands together. Parents and caregivers need to know how to use the child's preferred unique prompts that improve the child's attention and coordination at the same time. Because personal hygiene is such a sensory-intense category of self-care, the same teaching techniques for teaching reading may not work to develop these skills.

Wiping skills (yes, we need to talk about it!)

Wiping completely and efficiently after urination or a bowel movement is a tricky skill to teach kids. They can't see much of what their hands are doing (or see anything at all!) as they manipulate the toilet paper or wipes. Cleaning their body without touching urine or feces is necessary to prevent a mess. For a child who struggles with coordination, attention, and sensory processing (especially the skills of sensing body position and touch pressure without vision), this can be a greater challenge than learning the signs of elimination urgency. Low muscle tone reduces proprioceptive registration and processing. It doesn't take much loss of sensory processing to affect wiping skills.

One way to assess a child's potential wiping skills is to ask them to sit at the table and wipe something sticky off a plastic plate. They can see the mess, they could be familiar with the food (honey and peanut butter are good choices), and they have the postural support of the chair and the table. A child with low muscle tone that displays good hand skills and attention might be able to easily learn how to wipe after elimination. This activity can be short, and it can be presented as a game rather than an evaluation.

Wiping activities might need to be repeated to help a sensory-averse kids build their tolerance and confidence before asking them to wipe their body. Practicing this exercise with wet wipes or toilet paper also develops familiarity with hygiene tools. Toilet paper is thinner than a wipe, and both toilet paper and personal wipes have different textures than a paper towel or a washcloth. A child who is new to wiping after elimination can practice with simulated wiping of their body (review the "dry run" technique from Chapter 6). Pretending to wipe while wearing clothes allows a child to practice the hand movements and the necessary postural control without getting chilly or accidentally soiling their hands or clothes. It can be repeated many times in practice to refine these movements. Advancing to "dry run" practicing with clothes positioned for toileting (pushed down or held up) adds to the challenge without the area being wet or soiled. Giving kids the simplest explanation for how to successfully wipe after a bowel movement is usually the best.

Wipe until your wiping comes back clean.

This works for many kids: Wipe once. Check the toilet paper/wipe. Wipe again. If they wipe a second time and the toilet paper has no feces on it, they are done. Time to flush and wash. If it is not, they need to wipe again. After the second wipe, and sometimes the first wipe, most kids need to flush to avoid clogging the toilet. Children learning to wipe frequently use excessive toilet paper or wipes. Counting out the sheets before wiping and creating a limit on the number of sheets/squares prevents excess and plumbing disasters.

Every child remembers the plumbing disaster they caused!
Girls can wipe after urination in either a standing or sitting position. For girls with hypotonia, choosing the position for wiping after urination may come down to a matter of stability and accuracy. Select the position where they can control their hand use without sacrificing their balance. If a child is unstable, they don't devote 100% of attention and coordination to wiping. An unstable child is also not able to use sufficient force when wiping. This may leave some stool or urine on their skin. It could be necessary to allow a very unstable child hold onto a firm surface with one hand while wiping with the other hand. Holding onto a caregiver instead doesn't promote independence. It creates a false sense of security. Girls should always be taught to wipe from front to back after urination to reduce the risk of a urinary tract infection. A girl that is very distractible or struggles to remember a specific sequence can use and up-and-down patting movement.

Maggie decided that Bella needed to practice wiping after peeing. It seemed like it would be easier to start there. Bella enjoyed playing with toilet tissue, tearing it into tiny little pieces that stuck to her shoes, Maggie's shoes, and anyone else's shoes that was unfortunate enough to use a bathroom after Bella. Maggie grabbed some flushable wipes (harder for her granddaughter to shred). She wiped Bella, choosing the up-and-down movement, saying "pat-pat" as she did so.

Amazingly, Bella repeated it. Well, sort of. "Pa-pa" was what she said. "Close enough" Maggie decided. Because her granddaughter had no way of telling <u>anyone</u> if she had a urinary infection until it was bad, Maggie thought this wiping method had a chance of reducing the visits to pediatric urgent care. Getting a urine sample from her granddaughter was only one part of the full nightmare of urgent care visits. "It would be amazing if I could be the one to solve this problem." Maggie felt like Florence Nightingale.

Wet wipes or TP?

The choice of what material to use for wiping often comes down to what is available, what a child can control best, and how safely it can be disposed. Some children must learn to use toilet paper because it is the most common choice at school and out in public. They are confused or distressed when they are required to change the materials they need to use for toileting in different settings. Other kids cannot resist using too many wipes; they run through a container of flushable wipes in a single day. This is a very expensive way to get clean! And still other children need to flush away anything they soil. Toilet paper is the safest choice for most household plumbing. "Flushable" wipes are known to create blockages in all but the sturdiest plumbing. They are almost impossible for septic systems to handle. This means that any used wet wipes need to be promptly bagged up and tossed out in the trash. Children learning to wipe with toilet paper often benefit from using a thicker and gently textured toilet paper in toilet training. Little fingers will not go through thicker paper as quickly, and some thick papers are lightly textured. This texture wipes skin slightly more effectively when a child uses the same degree of force or control. Some toilet papers marketed as "soft" are also strong and slightly textured. Two U.S. toilet paper choices that work well are *Cottonelle UltraComfort Care and Charmin UltraStrong.*

Larger wet wipes can be very handy at the beginning of training. They are thicker and softer than standard toilet paper. The ***Dude Wipes*** brand is widely available online and in stores around the U.S. Wet wipes help children with limited grasp and coordination control their movements more effectively. They increase the amount of sensory feedback due to texture and moisture, aiding a child who has poor perception of force and touch. Wipes marketed for children have charming graphics, but the wipes are not always identical in size to the standard flushable wipe. If a child is over 5 or large for their age, they may need the larger wipe for full coverage.

Flushing the toilet

Flushing the adult toilet can be physically difficult for some children with low muscle tone. It takes a level of hand and wrist strength and grasp stability to fully depress the lever or the button with one hand. Toilet handles aren't always located in the best location for easy and accurate reach. Due to a child's smaller size, they are often reaching up to chest height and trying to deliver a downward force at an awkward angle.

James was eager to flush the toilet, but he was so short and unsteady that he had to use both hands to push the level down all the way. Lewis thought of putting a footstool next to the toilet, but then he imagined that doing so would be an invitation to climb on top of the toilet. "Well,", he mused, "The one thing I know is the kid will get taller. He is already curious. I don't want to hear that footstool scrape along the floor and discover him reaching over the stove to get something."

A child might be able to stand on a footstool to achieve better leverage. It is fine for an adult to help them initially, but how assistance is provided matters. Adults should avoid placing their hands over the child's hands. This type of "hand-over-hand" assistance reduces a hypotonic child's ability to sense the true level of force needed. It diminishes neurological feedback from their efforts. Simply put, "hand-over-hand" assistance placed on a child's hand slows learning due to a decrease in essential sensory information loops. An adult that wants to help a child flush should steady the child's wrist or forearm and allow them to hold the handle instead.

Washing hands after using the potty

Washing hands after toileting is an important hygiene skill. Some children will be experts in hand washing from their practice at school or during targeted pre-training. Other kids aren't as skilled. They assume that their caregivers will still take over some parts of hand washing after they use the toilet. And so do many parents and teachers; they don't see this as a toileting skill. At least, not yet. This makes hand washing a commonly incomplete skill well into formal toilet training. A child with low muscle tone may be able to get the soap on their hands and play in the water, but they don't wash and dry their hands independently. Ideally, developing independent hand washing AND drying is a pre-training skill. But if a child has already started formal potty training, they need to learn how to wash and dry at the same time as learning to use the toilet. Children will always need to wash their hands after peeing, as well as washing before and after they eat. This means that are many daily opportunities to build this skill.

The right soap choice could improve initial interest in hand washing, or it could boost waning interest as this skill is progressively mastered. Foaming soap tends to be more interesting to children and much easier to handle than the use of bar soap. Dispensers that have a large base are more stable, and pumps that are moderately easy to press prevent the container from slipping away from a child that is only using one hand (or weakly using two!) Scented soap can be appealing, or too stimulating, or very distressing; it all depends on the child's sensory issues. Some soaps are more entertaining than others. **Splatz** soap beads pop open when squeezed. This can give a motivational boost to a child who learned to wash their hands and is now blasé about the task. **Splatz** are not edible, meaning that their use must be restricted based on a child's safety awareness.

Henry's teacher was thrilled that Jordan wanted her to work on hand washing at school. "We have it as a goal in his IEP!" was what she said the minute Jordan mentioned it. "Who knew?", thought Jordan. That IEP meeting had been a blur, and the original paperwork was deep in a pile of paperwork, on top of another pile of paper, in her ex-husband's home office. There was never any time to read and file it all.

The teacher didn't want her to send any materials into school, even though that was one of the ideas Jordan read online. Henry was big on Paw Patrol, and she had scored a pump soap with a container covered in Paw Patrol graphics. Jordan nearly cried when she saw it on the shelf in the store. But the teacher mentioned something about protocols and rules, so she dropped this idea. She would keep it for home use.

Jordan knew her son's negative reactions to scratchy fabrics. Her mind went to the rough paper towels in the school's bathrooms. She decided that she could pick up some similar towels at Costco and start using them at home. If she couldn't get them to replicate what she did at home, she would try to copy them and help him get used to using scratchy paper towels. It wouldn't be very hard to try. The other things in her life were a lot more work than making another Costco run.

Some kids without sensory processing issues resist hand washing because they have learned to wash their hands only when they are visibly dirty. It seems like a waste of time to them. Hand washing is taught to follow or precede specific actions in addition to being done to clean off a visible mess. It needs to become a healthy habit, not an optional action.

For every child that dislikes hand washing, there are an equal number of kids who cannot wait to get wet and soapy. Once a shirt is soaked or a floor is flooded too many times, even the most tolerant parent will want to reign this in. If water and soap play are excessive and having to clean things up is not a deterrent, switching to use of a wet wipe or hand sanitizer is an appropriate response. Setting a clock-style or a musical timer helps children know when they are done. Kids who love water play need to identify something more desirable to do in another location to get them out of the bathroom.

Some kids have mastered washing up, but they don't dry their hands. A few weak contacts with a towel aren't enough to prevent soaking the next object or person they touch. Adults might assume that the child who walks away with wet hands is not trying hard enough to dry off. They might be surprised to learn that this child doesn't know how to use a towel correctly, or that they struggle with the two-handed coordination to get the job done. Better demonstration and more practice are the solutions. A larger towel, a smaller towel, or fewer distractions can help as well. Some kids don't know how to tell if their hands are still wet if they can't see water dripping off their fingers! They need experience and feedback. Placing the back of their hand on their cheek can be all the information they need. There are other ways to making hand drying more appealing. A towel with a desirable color or graphic can be motivating. Decorated disposable guest towels are sized right for smaller hands. Having their own special hand towel is also a way to motivate the reluctant hand dryer.

James had finally mastered washing his hands at home. He was clearly proud of not needed anyone's help. So was Tiffany. Telling Jacqueline and his teacher, Zulema, felt great. Sending Zulema the video of his skills felt even better. Tiffany wanted her to know she wasn't over-reaching or exaggerating when she reported this success. Switching to unscented foaming soap worked, as did cheap foam floor padding against some of the walls and buying a huge super-absorbent bathmat on the floor directly in front of the sink to absorb splashes. The foam padding was easy to sanitize.

She had tried using the foam mats in front of the sink, but there was so much water on the floor after hand washing that the matting made it unsafe. She grabbed two extra bathmats at the store. This allowed her to wash one at a time, and there was always a dry spare if he decided to go wild with unsupervised water play. Tiffany was confident that her plan to reward James for finishing before the 20-second musical timer ended would end that splashing.

Cathy Collyer, OTR, LMT

Chapter 12

Bumps in the Road

Smooth sailing through every step of pre-training and formal training is the hope and the dream of every parent and every professional that begins potty training. Even when they know the challenges that exist, the dream of seamless learning and rapid results can persist. To achieve the dream, there must be a plan to effectively deal with the problems that crop up along the way. Unfortunately, not every problem can be anticipated. Children are not totally predictable creatures. Schools and other adults can respond in completely unexpected ways. There will almost certainly be a few "bumps in the road" for every family on the way to toileting independence. This chapter describes the most frequently encountered challenges and offers practical strategies to help get things back on track.

Setbacks are not always crises. It can certainly feel that way on a rough day. Having a child with significant hypotonia could set a parent's stress level to "high" on an average day. It can be difficult to ever feel relaxed enough to calmly parse the difference between a small issue and a big issue. This can be true for their teachers or their therapists as well. Doing a great job doesn't mean that it is easy. Being humble and being willing to work as a team are hallmarks of a seasoned professional. Asking the rest of a child's team for help or feedback provides a different perspective. Grandparents have some experience in this arena; we know that they have raised and/or potty-trained kids before.

Should we take a total break?

What if pre-training or formal training needs to pause? There can be good reasons to temporarily stop toilet training. They come with risks, even if they are excellent reasons. The risks are more than simply increasing the total time to fully train. Kids don't understand that their parent is on a business trip, or that their nanny suddenly returned to her homeland. Lapses in expectations message to the child that what was important to adults is no longer as important now. Thinking that you need a break isn't a character flaw. It is the predictable response to having too little time and energy, and too many accidents, all the time. This is one benefit of using this book before beginning potty training; knowing the terrain ahead can make it easier to create a good plan.

If a parent is absent due to illness or employment needs, the remaining adults present tighten their focus on routines and rewards. Almost all children find familiarity reassuring when other parts of their life changes. When their routines are maintained, it keeps a child's skills sharp. Learning usually speeds up when more adults participate in pre-training or formal training. A child that has learned the words for body parts and bathroom equipment needs to use them in as many aspects of daily life as possible, and with as many people as possible. New skills should always be incorporated into a babysitter's or grandparent's expectations unless there is a good reason not to do so. During a necessary break in training, this becomes more important than ever before. A necessary break includes a child's hospitalization or severe illness, a vacation without proper equipment, and another type of training intensive.

New digestive issues

Constipation and/or diarrhea can come out of nowhere and occur in the middle of training. The most common causes are illness, diet changes, and emotional upsets. These conditions need to be handled quickly to avoid the risk of upsetting toilet training. Chronic constipation or diarrhea that starts in the middle of training can result in resistance or avoidance around anything to do with elimination. Kids with new and persistent digestive issues might begin to think that the diaper is the only familiar and safe choice. Allergies and food sensitivities could crop up. New classrooms might switch out snacks or beverages. A new food texture or an illness that caused a period of vomiting or other temporary digestive issues could take potty training off-track.
Returning to pre-training or formal training and a familiar schedule needs to happen as soon as possible. Children need empathy for their recent discom-

fort, but also assurance that things either will get better or visible and repeated demonstration that they already have improved. If they balk at using the toilet they get better incentives, while adults are both emotionally warm and firm about expectations. Children who have lost ground due to a break that is managed well may catch up quickly.

Managing the most common bumps in the road

The untrained child has been eliminating into a diaper since the day they were born. Toilets might be a new experience, and the concept that they should use the toilet instead could be completely unfamiliar and frightening to them! Novelty of any kind can produce fear in children with cautious temperaments or kids who have a history of failure and struggle. And most kids realize very early on that they could fail often without that diaper. Diaper use doesn't require skill, targeted attention, or action. It is familiar and foolproof. Along with not being comfortable with novelty, there is the unpredictability of having an accident. Accidents are just that: they are unexpected events. Placing a negative judgment on accidents is how kids decide that they have failed instead of simply making an error. While most adults realize that intentionally shaming a child is a mistake, the older child with low muscle tone can independently develop inherent feelings of shame. Younger children do not have the mental capacity to form these thoughts.

An adult's reaction to an accident needs to be nuanced and specific to the child and to the situation. During Collaborative Diapering and targeted pre-training, parents, therapists, and teachers have learned a great deal about a child's strengths and needs. Formal potty training is the time to put that knowledge into action. Kids who are profoundly averse to failure sometimes decide that they would rather choose to fail than to try and have the same outcome. This is simple and quite understandable; *if they aren't trying, they also aren't failing.* This is the classic underachiever stance. The only difference is that it happens in the bathroom, not the classroom or the office! Giving the failure-averse child the greatest chance of success means giving them the skills and the environment to succeed, and reacting to challenges mindfully.

Addressing fear of failure is best done by making it clear that accidents are not a big deal to the adult helping to clean them up; they are even expected when anyone is learning a new skill. What is important is recognizing, out loud, that the child tried to sense and respond to their elimination cues. Identifying what skills are missing and teaching them effectively will make a huge difference.

True accidents are chances for both kids and their caregivers to figure out what went wrong and possibly to adjust their plan. Adults that model the emotional management of frustration and disappointment provide a blueprint for children to learn how to handle their fear of failure and the disappointment of accidents. Of course, if it wasn't an accident, the response will change slightly.

Because of their immaturity, kids can have fears that would never occur to an adult. Children can perceive the elimination of stool as the loss of a part of themselves. They hear the stool splash into the toilet. Children aren't operating on pure logic. Magical thinking lasts longer in some children than others. The greater focus on elimination in potty training creates greater awareness of the release of stool from their body. If they believe that it is a part of their body, that can be frightening. Children need to be assured that their complaints are heard, whether they are real or otherwise. Knowing that it is not part of them, that it is the part of their meals that their body doesn't want to keep, makes it easier for some kids to let go.

Children who are more physically relaxed and confident are less fearful of being on the toilet and eliminating. Conversely, a child that feels unstable and is fearful of falling would be understandably avoidant of sitting on the potty. Those kids need a more stable or more comfortable toilet seat insert, or the addition of a footstool. Fear is also a common reaction to being overwhelmed by sensory input. Adaptations in the bathroom which reduce sensory stimulation and improve sensory modulation should be used. It is not essential to quiz the child on their fears, as many kids struggle with insight. They could know the source of their fears, or they could parrot back something they heard another child say, or something they heard an adult say about them. Targeted pre-training and collaboration with a child's occupational therapist could be incredibly helpful in addressing many of the most common fears that arise during formal toilet training.

James was making real improvements in all his toileting skills, but he was so short and unsteady that he still had a lot of fear when he was turning to sit, as well as while he was sitting to poop. Lewis thought of placing his hand on his son's shoulder to steady him, but then he decided that doing so would make it seem to James that it could teach him that having an adult with him was the only way to be safe. There had to be another way to make sure that his son could BE safe and could FEEL safe. Lewis saw how the progress they had made could evaporate if James decided to insist on a diaper. He thought hard. "Well,", he mused, "The one thing I could do would be to switch up our equipment. I saw something on TV about how a textured grab bar can also have a part that holds the toilet paper roll. I can install that myself."

Withholding urine or feces can come from defiance. The defiant child often enjoys the control they have over adults, including negotiating cooperation to receive a better treat. Once a defiant kid no longer receives attention for being defiant or loses their chance for any reward by stalling in the bathroom, the behavior might end after they recover from the shock of experiencing real consequences.

Children who withhold may not be defiant. They are consciously withholding pee and poop, and they have the physical control to "hold it". Common reasons for withholding are struggles after illness, due to fears, when a child perceives being judged for having an accident, or when a child feels a loss of control in another aspect of their daily lives. They often will use the toilet later, or in another location. Older kids may want privacy but do not know how to ask for it or may not be aware that they can request privacy. Until now, they have been accompanied every single time they have tried to "go". It is time to give those kids some space. Some children do not want to use the toilet in an unfamiliar place, and some children refuse to use the toilet without a parent nearby for emotional or physical support if they end up needing help. Discovering if any of these common issues are contributing to withholding behaviors is essential. Unfortunately, most young children don't calculate how long they can wait before they have an accident or become constipated. They will have frequent accidents or develop constipation or bladder infections. These can increase fears and emotional turmoil around toilet training.

Kids who have had problems with constipation and diarrhea may avoid elimination to avoid pain or embarrassment. Withholding can also happen if a child needs assistance for clothing management or wiping and isn't comfortable asking the babysitter or any adult other than a parent. Shy children may not express this discomfort; they may just insist on a diaper or refuse to eliminate. Children that have had a urinary tract infection or a stomach virus after they started toilet training can consciously or unconsciously associate potty training with the illness. Some older kids want privacy for elimination, but do not have the ability to identify that need. Voluntary withholding has consequences. The pee and poop are going to come out eventually. This usually means accidents, because most children cannot anticipate and respond effectively when they realize that they can no longer withhold, and they must eliminate. In addition to accidents, children can develop urinary tract infections due to the infrequent emptying of the bladder. There is a condition known as "lazy bladder". This results from persistently withholding urine. It is often accompanied by recurrent bladder infections. Chronically withholding urine overstretches the muscular bladder wall; the embedded nerves no longer trigger the urge to urinate. This can become a serious medical problem if it is not addressed. Withholding feces creates hard masses that are much more difficult and more painful to eliminate. It is a self-perpetuating cycle. Chronic withholding of feces can affect the natural motility of the intestines. Pediatricians and other medical professionals should determine if medical as well as behavioral strategies are needed to help a child end a withholding cycle.

Should defiant or withholding kids wear a diaper? It depends on the child. Some parents do not allow this. They are prepared for the mess and have restricted a child's access to spaces in their home that can be easily cleaned. Other parents put a training diaper on their child and change them without eye contact, conversation, and do not place a consequence on using a diaper. For a child that enjoyed being begged, pleaded with, and cajoled, this severely reduces the attention they crave. Kids that have intentional accidents are either expressing their emotions through an action or are using it to receive negative attention. A final word about using physical punishment for intentional accidents and defiance. It just doesn't work out in the long run.

Knowing where the closest toilet is located and being able to get to the toilet in time can make all the difference between success and an accident. Adults do not realize that they automatically assess their surroundings and anticipate their future toileting needs in unfamiliar environments. Noting public signs for the bathroom and recognizing that a closed door in a hallway is likely to be a powder room happen without conscious thought. Children are too inexperienced to think in advance about their bathroom needs and judge how long it could take them to get to a bathroom. Combined with the more sudden development of elimination urgency created by having a smaller bladder than an adult and less refined sensory discrimination, the child who is too far from a bathroom when "nature calls" is a high risk for an accident.

Parents and caregivers can point out the location of the nearest bathroom and make using it more routine rather than depend on a recently trained child to bear the executive functioning burden. Taking a child to a location without convenient access to a bathroom can result in having to pull the car over onto the shoulder, carrying the child at a trot to the bathroom, or cleaning up a puddle in the middle of their mother-in-law's living room!

Motivators, also known as rewards, can change as kids build their toileting skills or as they age. Very young children are more motivated by adult praise than children over 4. Still older kids are highly motivated by being seen like their peers or older siblings. Older kids may respond better to social motivators. Being compared to older siblings or relatives can be more exciting than copying mom or dad. If toileting routines have been flexible, tightening them so that there is no question about using the toilet before or after an event can help. Potty use isn't related to rewards at all; it is just a part of getting ready for school or for the park.

Consequences are harder to implement. They should be natural consequences if possible. Natural consequences are when a child's actions naturally result in a negative result for them. Having to stop all play, clean whatever was soiled by their accident, then strip down and take a bath without toys (only to wash their body) is a natural consequence. All this time may cancel out something they wanted to do. Because an adult is supervising, the time they would have been able to use for "x" is gone. The consequence is that the child loses something they care about, as well as the adult.

Loss of motivation are common responses once the novelty of using the toilet

151

has worn off. Using the toilet is just one more boring need that takes them away from playing or socializing. We see this with using forks and spoons as well. A child who perceives using the toilet as optional, and accidents as low-cost choices that allow them to keep playing, is going to have more accidents with less active effort to stop them. Loss of motivation to use the toilet occurs more often with older children who are beyond the age where pleasing adults is very rewarding.

Turning around the loss of motivation without immediately creating more punitive consequences requires adults to first reassess what motivates this child at this point in time. Refusal to use the toilet after initial mastery is common when a child feels powerless to control their environment. Children who seek control are aware of the power their refusal has on others. This can be resolved without breaking a child's spirit.

Henry's teacher was aware that his early enthusiasm over peeing in the toilet was waning. Fast. She knew if she didn't come up with a strong new motivator, there would be a good chance that he would not get up when he needed to "go". Henry was developing an interest in playing with one of the boys in his class. Whatever Keelan was into, Henry made sure that he was in the middle of it too.

The next time Keelan was taken to the bathroom in a small group, she included Henry. And she praised Keelan from here until next Thursday. He grinned and high-5'd her. She got him to high-5 Henry, and Henry was thrilled to be included. Then after Henry used the bathroom, she got Keelan to give Henry a high-5. This was all reported in the communication book that went home with him. Everybody at home needed to mention his new bestie and his new bestie's skill in the bathroom!

Defiance is different from fears. Defiant children often have a pattern of defiance in other aspects of their lives. It wears down parents' patience and can negatively affect the parent-child relationship. Children who choose to defy an adult's prompts to use the toilet or to perform the steps of using the toilet can be struggling with some aspect of toileting but are unable or unwilling to talk about them. It is not uncommon for the desire for privacy to be a reason for defiance. Too many accidents may have discouraged them, but they don't know it. All they know is that they don't want to think about, speak about, or be involved in toileting. When providing opportunities for emotional connection and successful independence in other areas of life make no difference in defiance around toileting, it is time to reassess a child's health and pre-training skills. The next step is to raise the desirability of motivators, perhaps with the child's input. An older child may be able to identify a highly desirable motivator that no adult has offered or even realized would work! A child that refused to go to the bathroom when told to (not asked, necessarily!) and then had an accident needs a consequence that is not punishment. They will be told that their accident was the result of their poor choice, but words, as they say, are cheap. This is when having to clean themselves up with a bit of help, and clean up any mess they can manage safely, sends home the message about choices and consequences. Some kids don't feel the impact of their choices unless the loss they incur is more meaningful. Having to miss a show that is left to run on a screen instead of paused, or leaving the backyard fun for a longer time, could make more of an impression on a child than having to take a quick bath.

The reasons for fears, withholding, defiance and disinterest change over time. Most parents and teachers know which kind of kid they have. Being able to pivot through the journey of toilet training isn't always easy for adults that use an authoritarian approach. Being able to place consequences on behavior can be uncomfortable for parents that use a "hands-off" style. It is always far more enjoyable to provide a reward than to implement a consequence. Almost everyone is better at consistently rewarding success than consistently carrying out a consequence. Successful toilet training when "bumps in the road" arise requires that the adults involved become skilled at both responses. The focus remains on skill building and connecting the dots between mastery and self-confidence, right through until the final step of toilet training: independent use of the public toilet.

Chapter 13

The Transition to Completely Independent Toileting

Most children with low muscle tone eventually become completely independent in toileting. The definition of "complete independence" is a child can use a bathroom alone, in any location, and at any time of the day. Bringing a porta-potty or a spare change of clothing along for family outings is finally over. Restricting their participation in social activities to a specific relative's homes or only using certain restaurants is done. They are dry during the night, all night because they can get to the toilet by themselves if they need to without being woken up.

This level of independence may take far longer than anyone expects. That doesn't mean that toilet training was done incorrectly or that a child has undiagnosed problems that require professional treatment. While those things could be true, it is more likely that their core training was adequate but incomplete.

This chapter describes how to work on nighttime dryness and how to build the skill of independently using the public toilet. Maintaining focus and motivation after the initial success of using the toilet in familiar daytime situations can be hard for everyone. Knowing what the challenges are, what the important skill sets are, and having practical strategies available make life easier. Too many toilet training books never touch these issues. That is unfair to the child with low muscle tone, for whom every success has been through hard work and determination. The hypotonic child deserves to have targeted training for this final stage that brings them to the true "finish line"!

Achieving nighttime dryness

A child who is successfully "day trained" at home or school can be slow to achieve full independent dryness at night. They may be using the bathroom alone, but still need an adult presence nearby for confidence or pre-use coaching. They may have a few accidents if they drank too much too late or were exceptionally exhausted by bedtime. This can continue well into elementary school years at home.

Most children without serious digestive issues do not have bowel movements at night; the brain automatically sends neurohormonal signals to the gut to dampen this activity. Achieving dryness at night is heavily dependent on physical maturation for both the ability to awaken when the bladder is full, and the ability of the bladder to both expand and retain urine. The mature brain secretes neurohormonal control to reduce the kidney's urine production at night. A child who has sleep apnea may not produce this hormone if they sleep too lightly; it is only produced during deeper sleep. A child who isn't sleeping well can be so exhausted that they can't fully awaken in time. Addressing and fixing the common causes of sleep apnea (obesity, enlarged adenoids/tonsils, asthma) and insomnia can speed up the development of nighttime continence.

For neurotypical kids, physical maturation for nighttime continence can be achieved anywhere from as early as 3 years of age up to 6 or 8. This final number sounds very late to parents who are tired of changing wet linens in the morning. Unless there are gut or sleep issues, it will be difficult to speed up physical readiness for nighttime continence. It is important to set children up for success. For the child with low muscle tone, that means making it as easy as possible to get to the bathroom safely, manage clothing efficiently, and reduce how full that bladder gets at night. It is helpful to limit any substantial drinks right before bedtime. There is no physical risk of doing this if a child has been well hydrated throughout the day. Eating dinner too close to bedtime damages the natural digestive rest period needed to induce and sustain sleep. Making certain that the child's path to the bathroom is clear of obstacles and ensuring enough light for walking there is essential. Pajamas and nightgowns that are quick to manipulate when half-awake should be worn. Kids can build some physical ability to retain urine by briefly delaying voiding during the day. They need to be wide awake and able to accurately sense elimination urgency. There can be few strong distractions that would weaken their attention and decision-making skills. Slightly stretching the bladder wall by delaying urination can only be done when a child is physically close to a toilet and are pros at managing clothing under time pressure.

The most surprising (and successful!) approach to building night dryness in a child that has the physical maturation is working hard on every daytime skill. Every. Single. One. A hypotonic child is less awake, thinking less clearly, and is less coordinated when they need the bathroom at 3 am. This means that if they still need help in the bathroom, reminders to be safe in the bathroom, or are used to ignoring urgency signals until an adult pushes them…they are in big trouble in the middle of the night. Efficient clothing management and safety while using the toilet are two that really matter at night. But the most important skill often isn't seen as a skill; it is seen as a personality quirk or a behavior. For the child with low muscle tone, it is as much a skill as a choice. It is the child's willingness to respond to their urgency cues right away. Any limitation in sensory processing reduces clear urgency signals. Combined with being half awake, the child who isn't consistently paying attention to their body's signals is going to have a lot of accidents. Adults who have been allowing them to keep playing until they are visibly uncomfortable and then insist the child goes to the bathroom have inadvertently been weakening a child's ability to sense and respond efficiently. The first step in building nighttime dryness could be allowing a child to have more accidents and teaching them that the responsibility for dryness is theirs now.

It is always preferable to reward a child than to place a consequence on their poor choices, but this would be one of the situations in which consequences make a difference. Rewards can include praise, just like during formal toilet training, but they can also be toys and experiences a child values. Bed alarms that buzz, vibrate, or ring can be helpful in waking a child who sleeps very deeply. They can also act as motivators since a child that finds them unpleasant could be more willing to get out of bed and avoid triggering the alarm. Extending the use of training pants at night beyond the point at which these are found to be dry almost all the time undermines a child's motivation to respond to their urgency cues.

Jordan and Lewis were so proud of Henry; he was using the toilet at home by himself! He still needed to get a few fish crackers as a reward, but he was doing everything alone, even washing and drying his hands. His wiping could be touch-and-go, but Lewis's sister said her own 4-year-old's wiping performance was no better than Henry's. What Henry couldn't do was tolerate using any other toilets, even with an adult helping out. Different faucets, a bigger bathroom, a smaller one; it didn't matter. He became so anxious that he would pee in his pants before he got them down around his ankles.

Using the toilet away from home or school

It can be a huge leap for a child to move from using their familiar and (possibly) custom-adapted bathrooms to use a public toilet. Some hypotonic children make this shift appear so easy that an adult could doubt these words. It seems effortless for them. That is, until a key aspect of their toileting routine changes with the environment, and they become very upset or refuse to use the bathroom at all. Parents and caregivers wanted to believe that all the hard work was done. Understanding that the goal of fully independent public toileting needs to be planned for, and that toilet training has an important second stage, is the path to success.

Without conscious preparation for the transition to public toileting, the consequences can be both surprising and difficult to overcome. Some kids are fearful of public toilets and become more resistant to toileting in general. An example would be a child who was not prepared to use the toilet at summer camp. The shock and fear set her back so far that she now insists on wearing diapers again at home. What was the difference between her home toilet and the potties at camp? The sounds and the unfamiliar space, without full privacy, were more challenging than anyone expected, and it overwhelmed her.

Begin Transitioning During Pre-Training, and Keep Moving Forward

Families can begin the process of transitioning to public toilet use by helping their child develop more independence when they visit family and close friends. This begins in the pre-training stage and continues through formal training and beyond. Even at the earliest stages, parents will be using all the pre-training techniques they have practiced at home. These include clothing management and hand washing in a bathroom. Because these homes are familiar, this should make generalizing skills easier. It is important to make sure that even if a child is wearing disposable training pants at grandma's house, they are changed in a bathroom. Pre-training principles require that the child is an active participant in the process of diapering. It still counts as progress if a child's only actions in an unfamiliar bathroom are to hold a fresh training pant or a wipe, and then flush the toilet. Becoming tolerant of the different sounds, smells, and sights in an unfamiliar but private bathroom will reduce overall stress when they need to use a shared bathroom in a mall or restaurant. Parents can take every opportunity to expose a child to public bathrooms by consistently using them to wash their hands while away from home instead of using hand sanitizer. Accompanying an adult or much older sibling while they use the public toilet also counts as exposure. This may require using the handicapped stall to fit two people inside.

During formal training, the use of unfamiliar bathrooms in family and friend's homes with adult assistance will be very important. Differences in equipment must be experienced, and any resistance or confusion overcome with warmth and exposure. If a child was used to finding the toilet paper on their left, it might now be on their right side. If their faucet at home was a single handle design, it is now two knobs for hot or cold water. How to get the correct temperature for hand washing should be demonstrated and explained. If they had a box of pop-up paper towels at home, they now need to use a cloth hand towel that goes back on the towel holder.

Bella was participating in every step of using the toilet at Maggie's house and at school with greater and greater skill every day. She remembered the entire routine and had very few accidents when she was taken to the toilet on schedule, and her diet and her health were both good. Getting better, in fact. Vacations from school and colds regularly destroyed her string of successes. Sean and Luke were still thrilled. She had made more progress in a short time than they could ever had expected. There had been very few tears, and no aggressive behavior at all.

A neurodivergent or very young hypotonic child may need a Potty Model for public bathrooms. In pre-training, Potty Models were used to introduce children to the experience of toileting in real time, with real people. Transitioning to using public toilets without being given ample opportunities to see someone perform the steps could be confusing for a child who struggles to generalize skills. The first step of Potty Modeling could be having the child observe an adult washing their hands in a public bathroom and looking at, but not using, the stall toilet. Smaller, less crowded public toilets are the ideal place to start. The local library or the toilet at an outpatient therapy center is a new potty in a familiar location.

Even if formal training at home and school is complete, kids may still need prompting or supervision when they are in an unfamiliar bathroom. They are not necessarily offered more assistance than they would at home unless it is essential. Offering the least amount of assistance possible to keep a child participating and calm will boost everyone's confidence and reinforce the message that independence is possible and expected.

Learning how to find a bathroom in an unfamiliar location seems simple. For a child that is taken from one therapy session to another activity, it is not. Pointing out the signs that indicate where bathrooms are located removes the mystery. So does learning how to ask a trusted adult to help them find a bathroom. An older child may feel self-conscious about how urgently they need to use the bathroom, but not know how to interrupt an adult to ask for directions or permission to leave the room. When the family enters a new restaurant or any new building, it can be a game to see who can spot the signs for the bathrooms first. At the very least, being explicit about the steps adults take to locate the bathrooms can decrease much of the anxiety that a child has about being fully responsible in a new environment.

James was fascinated by the bathroom at the elementary school his cousin attended. Tiffany and Corey had thought they would just play on the playground, but when his cousin needed to use the toilet, James decided that he had to go inside too! Instead of being afraid, he was enchanted to see more than one toilet. He flushed every toilet in the empty stalls, in order. The noise seemed overwhelming to Tiffany, but James handled it well. He left the bathroom grinning from ear to ear. "We will have to bring Will with us to every bathroom in town", thought Corey. The secret weapon for his son might be an older peer model.

If a child refuses to use an unfamiliar bathroom without adult accompaniment, the adult can be silent while helping them, using gestures rather than words to direct them through the steps. If a child refuses to manipulate their clothing, the first step in clothing management can be silently done for them. Once their pants are unfastened or slipped over their hips, many kids respond automatically and will continue to go through the steps to use the toilet successfully. Getting stuck at the initiation phase is a common problem with neurodivergent kids of all ages. The adult that is accompanying the child should gently acknowledge their success when using the bathroom or when walking out. Dramatic praise can trigger neurological activation in a stressed child, erasing the focus needed to complete all the steps in the toileting process. It can also prevent them from calming down after a challenge.

Having the right equipment for using the community toilet

Parents who are ready to move their formally trained child into potty use outside their home need to revisit their travel diaper bag. It is time to stock it with slightly new supplies. It should include some of the same things they have always stashed inside: rash crème, at least one complete change of clothes, anti-bacterial cleaner, and a stain stick. They need to add an extra pair of underwear, training pants/diaper (in case a child balks at putting on underwear after a messy accident), and either some large-sized flushable wipes or thick toilet paper for confident cleaning.

The decision to use a folding seat insert in public is done on a situation-by-situation basis. While portable, these inserts can be very wobbly and difficult to fully sanitize outside of the home. They are mostly a transitional, and thus a temporary, solution for public toileting. Children physically grow out of them or will need an adult-sized seat insert. But when they work for a child, they really work. Introducing a new device in an unfamiliar setting is a recipe for a scene. An unpleasant scene for everyone. Even in the very best situations, this device will not feel as stable to a child as the larger solid insert or the toilet seat they use at home. It could frighten them enough to refuse to use it. Folding seat inserts should be test-driven at home and at a friend or relative's home before being used in a more public toilet. If a child is in a growth spurt, reintroducing a folding seat insert is a good idea before taking it on the road. It may not be needed. They could be large enough to sit on the adult-sized toilet.

161

Not all children will still need the support of a footstool when they are ready to use the public toilet. They may have grown larger or build more stability and safety. A child can place their feet on an adult's legs if needed: the adult becomes a temporary footstool. Folding footstools are another alternative, but they are another thing to lug around. Families should only consider bringing one if this is an essential item to prevent falling, screaming, or soiling. Some families leave their folding stool in their car.

Full Independence in Public

The social behaviors in a shared public bathroom are different than using the bathroom at home. How much eye contact or physical closeness is considered acceptable can be spelled out for a child that may be more focused on being able to sit on a higher toilet. Teaching every child about handling a stranger speaking to them or touching them in any way is important. In the intensity of working on sensory and motor skills, this aspect of using the public toilet can be lost or minimized. Children can follow simple guidelines and will appreciate simple strategies they can use if any stranger interacts with them. The time will come when a child is able to go into a public bathroom completely alone. They may balk at this if the silent presence of an adult has been their "insurance policy" if anything goes wrong. For a child like this, the adult can enter the bathroom with them and then leave to wait close by. Insisting that stalls are locked before use and never sharing a phone or personal information, regardless of what anyone says to them, are two essential strategies that send kids with low muscle tone into independent use of the public bathroom much safer.

Conclusion

Leaving diapers behind and only using the toilet is a huge developmental accomplishment for the hypotonic child and their family. This book has explained why low muscle tone creates so many challenges for kids in potty training. It has covered the skills needed as well as the approaches that make the process easier for them as well as for the adults that love and care for them. Families and professionals need and want simple information about the process, strategies that work, and support to make it through to the finish line.

Comprehensive preparation for every step is essential for successful toilet training. Preparing a child to learn this complex skill is simply the kindest thing that can be done. They are too young to comprehend the reasons why these skills are harder for them to master than their siblings or peers. Great equipment and solid teaching can overcome fear and resistance. I cannot emphasize enough how essential it is that the parents, caregivers, teachers, and therapists are prepared well. Adults will be acting as teachers and as coaches. Their enthusiasm and patience will set the tone for training. If they feel discouraged or frustrated, a child will have a hard time feeling confident.

Toilet training can happen in a few months, or it can take place over more than a year. It is a journey you take with a child. But it can be done.

Be well prepared, be consistent, expect to practice, and stay positive.

You can do it!

Readiness Checklist

How to Use the Checklist for Optimal Results

- Cross off each item that a child has already achieved.

- The remaining items are part of your pre-training or formal toilet training plan.

- Go for the "low-hanging fruit" first. This gives you a chance for early success; start strong to win! Complete training of any partially achieved skills.

- Request feedback and assistance from the child's treatment team for skills that concern you. They know the child and have a unique perspective to offer.

- Do <u>not</u> minimize the benefits of having optimal equipment, including clothing and wipes, for eliminating barriers to successful training.

- When a training plateau, regression, or new problems arise, review this list to identify any missed training opportunities.

<u>Toilet Training Readiness Checklist</u>

- *Is there room in the family budget for disposable or cloth training pants, wipes, and/or washcloths?*

- *Can clothing for training be purchased, borrowed, or made?*

- *Is there room in the budget for extra laundry?*

- *Can potty seats, toilet inserts, footstools, etc. be purchased or borrowed?*

- *Does the child wake up in the morning or from a nap with a dry diaper at least 3-4x/week?*

- *Is their diaper dry for at least 1.5-2 hours while awake?*

- *Are their bowel movements formed and pain-free?*

- *Can the child sit on a potty seat or toilet seat safely and independently without fear?*

- *Can the child tolerate the sounds of a toilet flushing, water flowing, fans running, and people speaking in the bathroom?*

- *Can the child remain calm and attentive while being diapered and dressed?*

- *Does the child recognize their name when called?*

- *Can the child follow a simple <u>familiar</u> instruction with only a brief verbal prompt or gesture? Example: An adult says, "Up, pull pants UP!" while tapping the waistband of a child's shorts. The child reaches for the waistband and wiggles it up an inch.*

- *Does the child communicate that they need a diaper change? Examples are bringing an adult a clean diaper, bringing the adult to the changing table, or pointing to their diaper before <u>or</u> after they pee or poop.*

- *Does the child understand words/signs/graphics for body parts and simple physical actions? Non-verbal indications of com-*

166

prehension would be touching the front of her diaper when asked if it is "wet" or standing up when an adult signs "Stand".

- *Can the child recall 2-3 steps to open a container or assemble a toy, even if they need physical assistance to accomplish it?*

- *Can a child recognize that the received a reward or praise because of their action?*
- *Can the child remember and anticipate simple daily routines at home or school?*

- *Can a child respond positively to praise or rewards?*

- *Is the child showing interest in independence in other self-care skills?*

- *Is the child interested in wearing underwear?*

- *Can a child wait briefly (at least 30 seconds) for a requested drink or toy?*

- *Does the child cooperate with simple requests more frequently than they become defiant?*

- *When a child spills food or breaks a toy, are they easily consoled and willing to try again?*

- *Can the child assist in any way during a diaper change?*

- *Can the child take off their pajamas or an unfastened coat?*

- *Will the child start to pull off their clothes to get into the bathtub?*

- *Has the child pulled off their hat and socks independently?*

- *Who will monitor diapers to learn elimination frequency and timing?*

- *Who will focus on menus, diet, and digestion?*

- *Is a child's schedule flexible enough for a "potty intensive"?*

- *Who will do the training during a "potty intensive"?*

- *Who will take over other household responsibilities during intensive training?*

- *Does the available equipment fit the child?*

- *Is the equipment sturdy and stable for sitting?*

- *Can the child place their feet flat on a footstool or on the floor while sitting or standing at the sink to wash their hands?*

- *Can the child get on and off the toilet independently or with supervision?*

- *Have bathroom hazards and distractions been removed?*

Made in the USA
Middletown, DE
21 March 2024

51873983R00096